HEALTH
WHISPERS

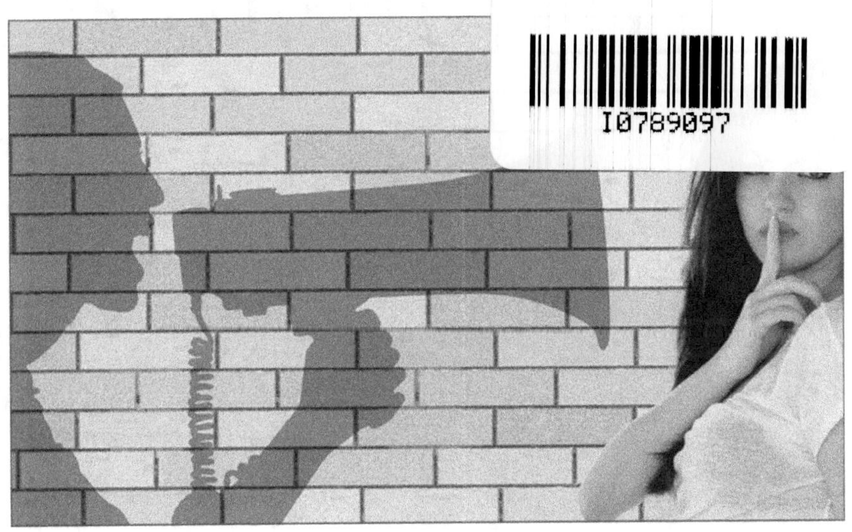

DON'T DIET, EAT RIGHT,
LOOSE WEIGHT AND FEEL GREAT, NATURES WAY,
while you still can IN THIS AGE OF MISINFORMATION
Quietly take back control

Healing from the Inside.
Stewart WHY

Disclaimers

This book is intended as a reference only, not a medical guide or manual.

The information herein is designed to help you make informed choices about your life and health. It is not intended as a substitute for any treatment prescribed by your doctor.

The program, recommended products and/or any other products and/or services and information offered here are provided to you on an "as is" and "as available" basis and all warranties, express and implied, are disclaimed to the fullest extent permissible pursuant to applicable law (including, but not limited to, the disclaimer of any warranties of merchantability, non-infringement of intellectual property and/or fitness for a particular purpose). In particular, but not as a limitation thereof, the publisher and/or health whispers makes no warranty that the information, the products and/or any other products and/or services offered herein: (a) will meet your requirements; (b) will be uninterrupted, timely, secure or error-free or that defects will be corrected; (c) will be free of viruses or other harmful components; (d) will have security methods employed that will be sufficient against interference with your enjoyment of the information and/or products, or against infringement; (e) will result in any specific health-related outcome; and/or (f) will be accurate or reliable. The website, the information, products and/or any other products and/or services offered within may contain errors, problems or other limitations.

Health whispers is not liable for the availability for the underlying interpretation, understanding, connection associated expressed or implied with any information, product and/or products and services within. No advice or information, whether oral or written, obtained by you from health whispers or otherwise through or from their associated websites and or other outlets, shall create any warranty whether or not expressly stated.

The information published in this book do not necessarily represent the ideas and opinions of the publisher.

Note: - This disclaimer has to be stated, as governments
everywhere have made laws about telling the truth that may be
against the stories of their beloved corporates and controllers.

Dedication

The information in this book was given to me, for you, I write and dedicate it to YOU.
I also dedicated it to my Dad who died early because of chemical usage in modern farming processes compounded by a catalogue of doctors mistakes in practicing their ideas on him like the old saying "being a guinea pig" and "Doctors don't really know what they are doing, they are just Practicing". To my Dad who showed by example that we must be interested in everything we possibly can be. And because I couldn't help him, it was for me to go on a search of discovery on health truths because it was clear he did not get any truth, just experimentation based around big Pharma thinking.

To my Dad who often stated that even those who are considered dull and boring should be listened to as they too have an interesting story if you can only bring it out. That if you cannot bring it out of them then it is you that is the dull and boring and uninteresting one.

To my Dad who understood about nature but got caught up in all the intensive farming concepts of his time only to say in the last few months of his life that those intensive ideas and practices were not only killing people, they are actually destroying the very land and environment we depend on for our food and therefore our survival.

To my Dad who through his loving we know love and through his strength we are strong. To my Mum who believed in the innocence of all, wherever they were in the world.

And to all the rest of the friends, the few family members and the victims of today's misinformation that have supported and experimented with me to prove the possibility of the truth of the information in this book.

To bring you an understanding of what Big Business does not want you to know And Politicians are afraid you will find out.

The stars may hold your destiny
But you have all the tools
Within you
To create it for yourself

CONTENT

Live without all that
Your money in your pocket
And your health in tact.

Do not be one that knows what to do
But does not do what they know

Tony Robins

1 ILLUMINATE

A little thought to Get started and knowing Why

This book and the information you find within is not just for you it is
for your whole family, your friends and colleagues too. It is not just
about losing weight but about starting real health for the rest of
your life.
Live by it and begin the feelgood feeling for as long as you live.
It is also about you and me with all our friends coming together as
ONE to stand for, demand and create a much better world.

Special Note:-
Statistics indicate that most people only read the first chapter of a
book they buy and if they get it for free it is never read.
Do not be one of those people with this book, read it all and
empower your own life and the ones you love too, for the better.

Be curious

> There is no point in making the journey
> any journey
> if you do not make every effort
> to find the truth and live it "on purpose".

It is of the utmost importance for you to have and to keep an open
mind while reading this book. Be open to writing a new history.
In fact, you must promise yourself that you will.
Then just observe your ego and feelings as you receive the
information within. Some of my friends have not and still suffer
unnecessary pain and discomfort as a result.
Your realities are generally defined by the people around you, and
by the regulations, misinformation and media which influence your
thinking, restrict your perceived options, and constrain your
creativity. You think you are "Right" with the information you have
but is it the right information to be "Right" about. As Tharv Eker
says in his money series "You can be Right, or You can be Rich"
the same applies to health and everything else in life. I say, "You

can be Right or you can be Healthy", "you can be right or you can be loved".
Or more correctly "You can Think you are Right"

An example, Are you enslaved to your dieting, type of food, bad information and bad habits that keep you hungry, unhappy and in your place and no matter how much you try to follow, you still put on the pounds, your metabolism is slow and all this makes everything healthy seem unachievable. Is this what you now believe, and do you really want this to be your "Right" information?

I say to you "Don't let that be your way or result", so when you find yourself rejecting an idea put forward here, stop and remind yourself of your promise to keep an open mind.

What are you being,
in the background of your mind
What is stopping you being, doing or achieving
that which you really want.

It is time for you to reconsider your position and decide whether you wish to continue supporting the present system at the expense of your own health, your freedom, your life and that of your children too or is it time for you to have and be something much better?

There is a large gap between "you" (the people) and the established industry and government information.
Compromise, contention, conflict and diversion are their tactics while money, power and control are their goal. In the absence of hope there is fear and uncertainty. Just as things are today. This brings certainty for their bottom line of their profit filled pockets.

Everything I write this book is stated in honesty and in trust. Not for conflict but with the best intentions to help you, your family and your friends to have a better life. The information here can empower you and your family to begin to take back control of your own health and lives. No more public lies and private truths or money stuffed shirts here, just the naked information.

> Truth is universal and you will know it
> when you see it, hear it or read it.
> For in truth you will find love
> Don't feel the love,
> no truth for you and me

I start therefore by stating that you should not believe a word of what you read in this book, as nothing you read in this book is true, well, at least according to the official line. You may also think that some of it is fiction but I do not have such a depraved mind to be able to make up what is being done in the world today. To the Human some of it is truly evil and crimes against you yet it is the truth that I have found to be behind the story you have been told for such a long time. Even those that are telling you these false stories believe their own lies for it is their truth in the interest of profit, power and control. Sadly, ALL is NOT as it seems to be.

> They have to maintain the narrative,
> because they are the dependable,
> of the shadow control over them.
> All bought off or blackmailed.
> When they can no longer be depended on
> to further the lies, they too become expendable.

Everything and I mean EVERYTHING is NOT as it seems to be.

> All is NOT as it seems to be
> Its time we all ask the hard questions
> Remove the darkness and Live in our truth
> Together, for WE are one.

THIS IS URGENT NOW. Please do your own discovery work and make your own decision. It's all out there and available to you if you question everything, dig DEEP enough, search far enough and you may need to read between the lines sometimes too.

> If what you Want, Lies buried.
> Dig and Dig and Dig, until you find it.

You have been informed or more correctly, misinformed throughout your life. Very little of what you are told is actually how it really is. SO, what must be considered about the Information you are told and then Questioned fully. Start by asking:
Is that information good for me (and for all of us, the people)?
also
Who is saying it and what is their agenda, what are they to gain?
Is that information good for them (big business, government),
Mercilessly masqueraded as the truth, Disguising their lies, money-making and control scams?

Remember it is better to gather your own information for positive and beneficial self-brain washing than to be trapped in today's Societies negative Programming where brain washing is so amazing, so effective, brain washed so clean, no thinking for self. If you do not or cannot believe what you read in this book then you have not done your own research and you remain woefully ignorant or you are a paid liar and part of the problem. Whichever it is I recommend you change your position and learn the truth about life here on this beautiful earth and how it can and must be. For if you do not stand with the people and the people fall, when they have finished with me they will come for you, your place is not safe.

> If you want a better world
> You must create and share a better story
> Of your own

Warning
Unfortunately the information at this time in history regarding health and almost everything else too is not positive happy or fulfilling, it is generally negative unhappy and definitely unfulfilling however it needs to be said and understood so the people of the world and you can get back to, and on with better things with joy in your life. Please be patient with me so you too can understand what to do for a better life of joy.

Because of the nature of things today this book may not be entertaining, although you may at first think it is fiction but it is not, or a simple or easy read as the information in it, although simple, may be confusing to those of you that are so misinformed with all the mixed messages constantly being put out there today. It is plain and simple, common sense, but complexity itself as common sense seems no longer to be very common, as common sense has been conditioned out of you throughout this age of misinformation where they think for you and tell you what is right or wrong to believe.

Fluff and fancy stories have been purposefully left out other than a few examples that may help you to get a better idea of what is portrayed and at stake for you. This is also a serious book about some of what you have been misinformed about and some of what you can do to correct what you have been, and still are, being misinformed about for the purpose of profit filled pockets, at your and my expense I might add.

Although some of the ideas put forward here you may consider amusing because they are so far out of the accepted conformed thinking, they are none the less as true as I can find, as you too will find if you do your own research. I am not a Doctor or trained medical professional so there is no real technical jargon. It also means that I am not enclosed or conditioned by those Label's and therefore have researched openly on myself and with many others to find the obvious and then experiment further with that truth through observation and intuition to find what answers your issues of today. Again and again I will say to you, Please do not just take my word for them, check for yourself.

Do not be disappointed if you are not entertained as there is so much information surrounding this subject that just the bare bones information is put forward here to introduce what is actually happening to you and to keep it as compact as possible for you so you have a starting point of understanding for your own research.

Having said that,

> There is no need to worry about the future
> as the future is already here
> full of love, truth and compassion.
> The controllers of today just don't know it yet

> But there is still work for you to do
> To bring it forth as quickly as possible
> From tyranny to freedom and liberty
> For all awake enough to grasp it
> Start, by demanding your leaders serve you
> Write to them daily if that is what it takes
> Then following the info passed to you in this book
> It will give you awareness and understanding,
> and ideas to look and feel your best,
> have better dreams
> and ways to live your life, on purpose
> prepare and become aware as fast as you can
> for the tsunami of change is drawing down the beach
> ready to wash aside the old into the archives of history.
> While the new story manifests with or without you
> What you do now will influence the outcome
> Why are you showing up here anyway
> To make some noise for good
> what will you choose to do, to become,
> to ensure it is a better world?

A reminder,
THIS IS URGENT NOW PLEASE GET ON IT.

Statistics indicate that most people only read the first chapter of a book they buy. Do not be one of those people with this book, read it all, act on what you find and empower your own life, read it several times and empower the ones you love for the better too.

> The process brings Motivation,
> Improvement,
> Joy,
> continue

2 DISTORT

Introduction to a world of misinformation and some Notes from the author

> You may say, "It's not my story so why should I care"
> You care because you are in the story anyway
> So it is your story too
> And that is why you must care

Today, there is a great gap between the people and their governments, between big business and their customers.
You are being betrayed in a big way.
Big Business and their puppet Governments, are all bought, manipulated and strong armed by anti-democratic elites which I call the Shadow Controller's that work behind the scenes. They have grown into huge beasts, working together against the people while you are taught to believe you are small and weak and all alone through fear mongering, separation, distraction and selfish ideologies, misinforming and strong arming you.

Our first big mistake is our silent agreement to them calling themselves the "ruling elite" and the "political class".
For they are neither of those things.

> The beast of power says, how can we control
> Coerce, conflict and compromise
> To bring fear through the absence of hope
> So we can prosper at the peoples expense?
>
> You and I must ask,
> how can we empower ourselves, each other
> Bring hope and understanding to the world
> And create a world that might just work
> Today is the time to break the patterns of past generations

> You are tasked to spread the word
> stand quietly with us and speak up when needed
> it's All about loving, Yourself.
> About living, Naturally.
> And about Why.
>
> No Money stuffed shirts and fancy ties
> or Private lies
> Just Naked Truth.
> In serving you
>
> The darkness of the past can no longer hide in the shadows
> Your light is bright, showing them for what they are
> pointing the bone and finding the cause
> whose plan are YOU working on anyway
>
> Thin whispers on the breeze
> Truth in the wind
> Now, rewrite the social contract
> power to the people, replenish the earth
>
> Learning develops you and eliminates errors
> keep up the pressure for power is accumulated
> live your own power in truth
> The Future is now

A reset of the social contract must happen but not the evil agenda 2030 the controllers have planned for you. Die billions die.
It must be a nature alignment with love and unity for one another.

Hello and Welcome,
They call me Stewart Why.
I want to thank you and commend you for taking action on your journey of life and especially your health. The information within was brough to me and is written for you, read it all and act on what you can. It is an honour to serve you and I embrace you with love and great health, for it is said

Life can change, Suddenly.
Out of all proportion, and without warning

This is very true of some things however not generally true regarding your health, except in some rare occasions it is usually years of offending your body that brings you bad health even when you think that this bad health came on rather suddenly. This means your ill health starts a long time before you see or notice any of the symptoms, feel it creeping up on you or have the real indication of it. You may be looking healthy on the outside while you are breaking down on the inside. This is not how nature works but it is the way things are today with all the manipulated and chemicalised food of today.

I was directed and encouraged to put this information together with the idea of giving benefit to you and those who not only read it but take action on the information within. There are many things in the book that I do not want to tell you as they are far from happy thoughts but until you realise what really is happening to you and everyone around you then we, together, collectively cannot put it right. We all need your light, your voice and your vote too, to reject what is happening and bring in a better way for us all. There is great danger for all humanity if the wrongs of the controllers are not stopped now for their plan will take us, you, me and humanity to the brink of extinction and a life of hell for those left behind.
It is not meant as a bashing of company or government, in fact I think we should all run our business affairs through a company or companies and some form of governance is necessary to manage the affairs of the people. This is not what we have today though as Companies and governments have grown into huge beasts with their respective controlling members addicted to power, control and money stuffed shirts. And you and I, the people, are just pawns to be pushed around at will and fleeced of every red cent and asset we work to achieve, bleed dry before being tossed aside.
 In fact, you may find some of the information within this book disconcerting and even heavy going but please stick with it so you get the full picture. The facts, ideas and thoughts put forward here

are purely for you to open your mind to what really is happening to you in the modern world, to help you to make better decisions. Again I say, Stats show that only the first chapter is read in most books, you will not get the benefits within if you do not read them all so I challenge you to not let that be you with this book, that you will continue to read and act on it all.

Here is just a brief coverage of my own health story so you know where I am coming from to bring you this.

When I was young, I used to think that I was invincible. I was also so fit I felt that I could easily jump over the moon without even much of a run-up.

I spent the first 20 years of my life preparing, and the next 25 plus years working and traveling and working some more to travel some more. I am not sure why I've been so obsessed with wanting to travel, perhaps to learn as much as I can from all the people around the world, their culture and way of life of all the places that I've travelled to. Almost 50% of the worlds countries and growing and I am thankful for every lasting and incredible experience and learning while connecting the consciousness net of earth protection. Blessed by such a purpose.

Among all that travel, some 35 years ago my father became ill and after much a to do with the so called professionals procrastinating and mismanaging everything relating to his condition and treatment they finally decided it was cancer and too late to do anything about it because with their actions they had actually spread it to many organs. In truth his condition was complicated by the series of serious mistakes by his doctors and the so-called specialists. Unfortunately, He became a real statistic of doctors burying their mistakes, literally........

I spent the last 7+ months of his life with him, supporting him and then nursing him. If you have not been through a situation like this you will not understand how distressing it can be, but if you have you will know the thoughts and feelings of wanting and wishing to be able to put it right so your family member did not have to go through what they were going through. It's not the dying, as sad as that may be, because we all know that at some point we will die. It is the knowledge deep inside of you, that somehow what is happening to them should not be this way.

So, with the thought above, I have since spent all of the 30 plus years in a quest to find some answers, sharing what I had to help those who would listen whenever I could along the way. This is now put together for you too to benefit, if you so choose it.
I had gathered much of the information but the answers did not become clear until a recent health crisis of my own.
It transpired that I did have much of the information but there remained a few small pieces missing to build a clear picture of the puzzle, and new information and new awareness still comes almost daily.
As you may know when you read up on a particular situation that the so-called authority's (or perhaps we should refer to them as the "official organizations" relating to your particular quest for information) have so many different things to say about the topic, which is confusing enough in itself, but also you may feel, that this information just doesn't feel right. It's impossible to put your finger on exactly why it doesn't feel right, so you just feel even more confused. At least this was how I felt for a long time until I learned to read between the lines or complete their sentences and look behind the story to reverse their speak to get their true message.
 Some of you however may just have followed or be following this information to the best of your ability and then wonder why health Is still no better or even deteriorating. When you talk to your doctor, they always have the standard throwaway quip "it's just a sign of your age" or some other similar worthless projection.
Whichever it is, confusion and sometimes frustration, along with ill health, are the end result.

My own health crisis started in 2000. While still feeling invincible, I was off to South America to climb mountains. The aim was to climb the highest volcanoes in the world. While there I got a very serious dose of food poisoning. I discovered afterwards that it was caused by cross-contamination of raw meat onto the cooked meat, so you too be careful of this. This was done by using the same tong's on the barbecue grill to remove the cooked meat from the grill to the big plate and then load fresh raw meat onto the grill and then use the same tong's just used on raw meet at the table to distribute the meat to our plates. Very simple mistake but make no mistake it can be deadly.

I spent 3 weeks extremely ill while my friends were off climbing mountains and I was just well enough to catch my flight back home. I slowly recovered and was starting to feel better again when almost 3 months later while at work I suddenly felt very tired. So tired that I had to sit. So tired that my legs felt like jelly. So tired that I couldn't think straight and my head and eyes felt as though they filled with a heavy foggy. This sudden change happened very quickly one morning and was more like a tsunami of sleepiness crashing over me than anything else I can describe it as.

In thinking about the situation, I can only explain it as driving along in your car and suddenly your car falters. You look down at the fuel gauge and you see it is below the "E" for enough, in fact it is so low that it is empty. The engine stops and things go silent. Unfortunately, you're going up a hill and the car slows rapidly and before you know it you are at a standstill. If you don't act quickly you will start to roll backwards down the hill but you are so sleepy you can hardly think of what to do next. In fact, the big slide down the dark hole of fatigue is now inevitable. This is exactly how it felt when the crisis struck me, I just ran out of fuel.

I endeavoured to return to work, resting for about an hour, working and hour. I muddled through like this through the next week at about 10% energy level because I had a project to complete. I rested, ate and slept for 3 or 4 days following this project in the hope to restore my health.

Remember prior to all this I was super fit and had as much energy myself as 3 strong men that never faltered.

There was little improvement from my days of rest and when I did return to activity my energy levels were back to about 10% after just a few hours. I repeated this process many times and still the same result. There seemed no way to refill the tank with some energy to function, I was always on empty and no way to build reserves.

Going off to the doctor to explain my situation and what was happening to me. The Doctor started to write a referral to a specialist that would help me. I asked him what this specialist did, and he replied" Oh he's a psychiatrist." So, I said to the doctor "I don't need a psychiatrist. A psychiatrist cannot help my body to restore its energy" The doctor in his stupidity said, "It is clear you have what is called fatigue and that is all in your mind." I thought

"What a fool" and then, "oh no, not a ""Label stuck on me"" " but more on that later.

Over time, having fatigue does do your head in with the frustration of it all, but at that time I was thinking clearly enough to know it was my body that needed help, not my mind.

Some people never get over fatigue and some even die, but that was not an option for me.

I have tried every remedy out there and more I made myself. I pushed and pushed and pushed to try and push myself through it. I would have a small gain, which plateaus for a while. Sometimes it slipped back a little and then I may have another small gain which plateaus. It is like trying to climb the mountain from a thousand miles away in very deep, small loose gravel.

After about 10 years of this, and some very difficult times I had gains and achievements to get my energy levels back to about 50% of my previous standard when I had another breakout of health issues.

I noticed when returning home on an international flight that my lower legs had become swollen. This was another 1st for me. What followed I would not wish on anyone. Over the next 2 years every joint and muscle in my body (and especially my legs) swelled, became extremely painful, and this pain travelled through my body from joint to joint and muscle to muscle like a giant python eating its way up one leg across my hips and down the other, then back again. Eventually the pain became so great that I was using 2 sticks to walk with. This was necessary because when the python bit and the stabbing pain struck in the legs it was most likely that I would have collapsed in a heap on the ground without them. I am still reasonably young, (although following the food poisoning my hair turned grey within 6 months or so) I did not want to walk with 2 sticks, so I got some walking poles to assist me. Even though I was trying to tell myself a better story and look like a fitness walker, I did need them for support and assistance when the pain struck me out of the blue. Another way to describe the pain was like having my own personal gangster by my side, moment by moment, stabbing me at random and without warning.

This frenzy of pain came to a climax one summer's day with the final reaction that had been building for many months. This reaction was unbelievable chest pains, feeling nauseous and the calling of the elite medical team. I am talking of the amazing ambulance people. They immediately considered I was having a heart attack and went through the process of supporting such a happening. I was admitted to hospital and 3 days later was discharged as definitely not a heart attack but health condition unknown. The doctor said, "All we know is that your heart is strong, you are not having a heart attack, but we do not know what is causing your condition."

One of the junior doctors made a quip as they left "It's time to stop pretending and get your butt back to work."

Now I've never been a pretender especially about ill health. I have been known to pretend that I am feeling much better than I am actually feeling but not the other way about. So, all I could do was go back to work, but my condition did not improve much.

After many more visits to various hospitals and specialists and countless rounds of tests of various kinds over the next two years or so I was told by the medical fraternity that they could find nothing wrong with me and that whatever was causing my condition was unknown. The 2 specialists at my final appointment said there was nothing more they could do for me and that I would just have to learn to live with it. And to top it off they said my state of health was in the hands of God.

Doctors usually say that to the terminally ill and I was not pleased to be hearing such nonsense from so-called professionals but that is how it goes now.

My work contract ended and I had some time on my hands before the next one so I started putting together all of the information that I had collected regarding health since my Dad had died because of his doctors mistakes and incompetence in the 1980s.

As I was not prepared to continue living with what was happening to me, it was not an option, I had to put every effort in to gathering and assembling the information for myself because it was very clear the modern medical profession and model wasn't going to help. After several weeks the jigsaw puzzle started to fit into place and a picture emerged. The basis of it is what I reveal here in this book.

I had been doing many of the principles discussed here but to bring my health to its state of crisis, there were some key exceptions that continued the deterioration of my body even though I had managed to improve my energy levels dramatically from the severe state of chronic fatigue.

Today I am grateful to say that I'm probably 95% returned to my former health and improving. So long as I stick to the food regime, I have set out for myself, this improvement continues. When I do not, I have the symptoms or indicators of my previous fatigue and more pain, taunting and jabbing at me within days and sometimes even within hours of straying. I changed doctors again and was referred to a gut specialist who discovered I had an ulcer and after a course of treatment I had another major jump in my health. If only the first doc had been more open minded to such a possibility it may have saved me 10 plus years of suffering.

What you read in this book is an overview of that understanding and some guidelines as to what you can do, to make your life a lot healthier and happier too.

This information has also brought results of better health for many of my friends and associates who suffer a variation of modern-day degenerative health issues, that have chosen to act on it.

It is with their encouragement and help that I have put pen to paper to put this book together, to help you too.

When you follow the concepts and tips in this book you will start to turn around your health issues whatever they be (either small or large). It will return you over time to feeling good. Over time, you may even be able to maximize the benefits of health improvements, contain or even correct some serious degenerative health issues, and reduce your fat levels dramatically if that is an issue for you.

Regain that feel good feeling like a younger person again.

Remember that the medical profession and big business do not want you to know (or do) this because when you are healthy there is no money in it for them. Remember also that nature works in a systematic way and therefore it will take time to do a proper repair. Unless you understand the power you hold within, there is no such thing as instant healing. Keep working at it because when you are healthy you hold the power of your own body.

And please help as many people as you can with this, by telling them to come and get this info for themselves.

Please spread the word discretely and speedily.

2 DISTORT

Perhaps now we should start with what each and every one of us can do to help each other, and ourselves and that is to work together on this. Only when working together do you and the rest of us have any real chance of success? However, if you do not have someone to agree to work with you on this, find someone or just do it on your own anyway.

It is the most important thing you will do for yourself
as the information can transform your health when applied.

No good just knowing it
because if you are not doing it
In reality, you do not know it at all

It is the action that will remove slowly so many of the unwanted toxins and gremlins that you are feeling daily in your body, to give you the knowledge and feeling of wellbeing in the near future.
When you take heed of the information within this book then I can assure you it is likely to change your life and health for the better.
Although I didn't just say all that did I?

Stay Strong and stay with it

Note to YOU:-

Until you have read all of this book,
It may not be all your fault

Is it fraud on their part
or innocence or even worse, ignorance on yours?
You decide once you have read this entire book.

The reality is,
Perhaps it is not all your fault
but it is your responsibility.

Before I go on I want to dispel the myth in your head that it is all a conspiracy theory. What is said in this book is no theory, it is fact as you will find if you are only open minded enough to research it yourself. There is a conspiracy though and it is against you and I and all the people of the world. Why do you think they created the idea of "It's a conspiracy theory" in the first place, because it is but you just got the direction of it mixed up. This too was created for you to reject anyone saying stuff out of the official narrative.

When I talk about "They" I am usually referring to the Shadow Controllers and their dependable's that keep up the story, pawns on their chess board to be discarded and crushed at any moment. For when the controllers have finished with you and me they will go to the dependable's and finish them next.

May I continue?

As you have been misled by/and for the benefit of the big corporations. They have taken responsibility to promote what makes money for their shareholders, but not to be responsible with what value, quality or even purity they promote to you, their customer. You do not matter to them other than the money in your pocket, they want it.

There are things that have been misguidedly put forward as truth initially sure, based on misunderstanding the information at the time or more correctly a lack of the full clarification of the information for a clear understanding of it. Then this information has then been taken and further manipulated for profit. Even when the information they have is found to be inconclusive or incorrect and the truth is then understood to be very different, their story is still maintained, distorted and manipulated for big business gains. To put it bluntly big business and their government puppets will bend any half-truth whether harmful to you or not for the money and power that they have become addicted to.

It is considered that as a rule that fat people eat far more than they need to and that fat is just excess calories of food energy stored as fat. There may be an inkling of true in this but what you are not told is that it is not so much of how much you eat that's important but how much of what you eat is the only important aspect to think about.

We have been lied to for years about so many things for the profits of the big business and the politicians. The low fat, high carb, processed food diets and super sizing meal deals with all of its toxins and poisons are just a few examples. There are many more to look out for.

If the world follows the present projected information accepted from the FDA of America and their ridiculous food pyramid, we will all be doomed to extremely poor health, little quality of life and for most an early death. Oh I almost forgot, that is in their plan for you

Some examples of their misinformation and myths.

Don't eat fat as you will get fat and clog your arteries
The first part is not true because as with all things all fats are not equal at all. Dead foods make you FAT but Fat itself does not make you FAT. Natural animal and those found in vegetables plus fats like cold pressed olive oil and coconut oil will not make you fat at all but all processed trans fats like vegetable oil, canola oil and all other oils that have been heat treated in their processing (including olive oil) although they too do not make you fat they will clog your arteries. The very opposite to what you have been told for years.

Doctors today are trained to look at the sick
in the hope they can keep you healthy
when surely it would be better to look at the healthy
to keep you from getting sick.

They are also trained to look at just one separate thing and to fix that one separate thing but surely nothing works like that as it is connected to the whole body system and therefore the effect of that one separate thing could be caused from elsewhere in the system. They are trained this way because it supports the big Phama narrative, for profit whatever the consequences. This was developed in the early 1900's and all the other health modalities' discredited on purpose so that they make the profit and you are the consequence who pays the price in every way.

Busting and correcting just a few of the myths

Virus, bacteria and fungus are the cause
Parasites, Bacteria and Fungus yes as they are living organisms that can clearly be observed but what are virus's? A virus is something that is said to spread fast like bill gates infecting all your computers or your post on SM spreading fast and wide. There is

much research that virus's thought to be observed in areas of the body that has been affected in some way, may not even exist outside the effects of the cells own process of repair. Now days some science research considers that what was seen may only be the aspects or fragments of dead cells being removed as the cells rearrange and change in the process of self-destruction and repair while the cause is something else entirely.

Could it really be microbial parasites or bacteria of some sort invading and attacking certain areas of your internal system and the fragments that are thought to be virus are just the fragments of dead cells being discarded. Or is it likely to be bad thinking affecting your body in ways as yet unknown with the influence of today's artificial and toxic chemical overload mixed with mutating bacteria or other affects on the cells from dead foods because it seems it is not what has been stated.

All calories are the same

How ridiculous is the idea that dieting is all about calories as one only has to look at the calorie charts to see that the calories in fructose may be a low 20 but are in truth extremely harmful to your body while the calories in parsnips and dates may be around 100 and yet they are both extremely good for your body. Just this little look is enough to tell you that calorie counting is a ridiculous way to being healthy. Forget the calories they serve no purpose in the process unless you want to be even more stressed than you probably are already.

Other myths but not just about calories:

Don't eat eggs as they will raise your cholesterol

All eggs and seeds are the essence of life and are extremely nutritious food. I have eaten at least two eggs and lots of nuts and seeds every day for 30 plus years and they help me to keep my cholesterol normal, stay slim and strong even through my health crisis and are a great source of protein. Unless you have an intolerance to them, eat them.

So, I repeat, it is most certainly, not all your fault.
But once you have read this book you will have no more excuses
And it really is your responsibility.

Important Note about food

It is important to note that one food strategy does not fit all. The food strategy set forth below is to those brought up in Western countries and those other countries that have adopted Western methods of food production and consumption.

For those living in different latitudes or localized areas with their own unique food types and consumption it is advisable to take note of the local food eaten and available. If your ethnic heritage is from one of these types or areas, then it is advisable to eat as close to the traditional food of that area. This does not mean necessarily, what they are eating today, as the traditional food may be diluted with imports of modern processed foods and ideas.

For example, a change to a Western Diet for the Eskimos would not have worked in the past as everything needed to be imported without the transport systems of today. It was necessary to live on the locally available food source of fish, seal meat and fat, and this is what they evolved to eat in their location.

Food considered healthy in the one area may be a disaster to the people elsewhere. The reason for this is that over many thousands of years people in all different parts of the world have developed distinct nutritional needs in response to climate, geography, and whatever plants or animals their local environment could offer and your genetic makeup has responded accordingly.

The same principal applies today. The people in different parts of the world still have different requirements regarding nutrition in the combinations of the primary and most essential building blocks of food i.e. proteins, carbohydrates and fats.

It is because we have changed our diets so rapidly (and even lightning speed for those who have travelled to live away from their origins in this lifetime) all in just the last 100 years. It is a flash in our history that our bodies are struggling to adapt to. It is documented that a migrant from a so called third world country is significantly healthier on arrival to the so called western or first world countries than the first world people around them Yet within a few short years they lose this advantage and sometimes drop into disadvantage as their new local people are . Their bodies needs are so depleted that they struggle to survive let along thrive. If this is you beware.

You just have to look at local eating around the world to see that traditionally in some areas there is a high meat content, others fish and others vegetables with little else included, so it is important to understand if possible your genetic or ethnic heritage and their traditional foods. In some places this may be difficult due to the genetic melting pot of multiculturalism. Where this is not possible it is a good possibility that you should start from the recommendations in this book and follow this process for at least a few months to work out your body needs. This will start the cleansing process and then add and/or adjust in small amounts until you find the levels of whichever foods that suits you most. This does not mean going back to your old diet but keep on the process set out below and adjusting the protein or natural carbohydrate content as explained. At the very least wherever you are and whatever your traditional food the chapters on "Removing the offenders," "Eating your Supporters" and "Fine tuning" are a must for all to follow.

Remember, if you have eaten shit for food for years to get this way and you want to take a pill to fix it. Nature does not work that way.

You may be able to speed this up with a water and green cleanse but in truth you will need to follow this process for at least 6 months, a full body cycle and more, for an initial cleaning process. Then each 3 to 6 months period following, you will have further cleansing and improvements. Once your body has removed enough of the toxins, the real rebuilding process will start.
Depending on how compromised you are, i.e. the longer you took to get here the longer it will take to clear up the mess so the longer you stick with this the better. Over time, your body will start to re-balance and even weight correction will likely take place.
It has at least, for those already doing this.
Listen to and feel your body, as it will tell you what is good for it and what is not.

If you have been eating poorly over the years, it may not be possible for you to understand your body message properly to be able to respond clearly at the start. It may also be confused in itself but give it a month or so and you will start to feel it indicate, "this is good" or "this is not".

When your body does start indicating what is good for it and/or what is not, then feel the reaction, take action and follow what it tells you.

Always remember that refined carbohydrate and sugar based, or laced foods always send the wrong signals to the brain see chapter on "Intolerance".

It is important to continue to do this at all times anyway as your body is a dynamic entity. That is to say it does not remain constant but change as much as possible to adapt to the changing environmental conditions. Your body has an inbuilt desire to achieve a healthy balance, to regulate itself in the direction of remaining healthy. Your need to change the foods you eat, may change from season to season, month to month. If you follow your biorhythms, you may get a better understanding of how your body changes and then a feeling of what you need to feed it. Hence the reason for targeting your traditional foods through the seasons.

When considering what is good for you to eat it is not just the foods of your genetic lineage, although this is a very important place to start, you must also consider the environment in which you live and the lifestyle that you lead now, as both of these may override some of our ancestral needs, especially if you are from the melting pot of multiculturalism.

In the last hundred years or so, a split second in evolutionary time, the essential qualities of your life i.e. our air, water, soil, food and environment have been profoundly and subtly altered. In reality, much of it has been ruthlessly altered in the name of profit on the pretence of benefit and now to justify it, blame it on global warming that we, the people, are responsible for. Another ridiculous and contrived concept that has been created on purpose but that is way to much for this book although some thought on this later.

It has been assessed that you are faced today with more than 1000 times the toxicity per day than your ancestors faced in a lifetime just a few generations ago. It is a miracle that we have been living longer today when you consider this, although this is also changing for the worse now. If one is to analyse the data, it may be considered that if our ancestors had the sanitation i.e. the clean water and waste removal of today, they may have lived to well over 100 years old in very good health. This is not even something we can boast today. At the moment we may live a little longer than before but there are two very important factors to consider here.

The quality of the last years of life in old age has been deteriorating rapidly over the last 30 plus years or so.
The kids of today are likely to die of ill health before their parents because they start life with dead foods and toxified environment. At least your grandparents started out eating live food.

A few more thoughts before we get on to the food. They are important to consider as they indicate why change is necessary.

It is strange to find that scientists have such difficulty in understanding, or more likely they know but just do not want to tell us because there is no money in it for them, why there are several primitive cultures living today that are almost completely free from all generative diseases that affect modern western civilizations.
Just this one fact alone clarifies who the misinformation/conspiracy really benefits.
It is clear from studies that when so called primitive cultures take up modern diets, they very quickly develop all the same chronic dis-eases they did not have on arrival that are so epidemic in modern western society today.
America claims to have the best health technology and methods in the world today yet have the lowest levels of the people's health, the world over.
The countries that have the biggest profits from drug sales and use the most intensive farming methods have the worst health record in direct relation to their implementation.
The higher the vaccination requirement of a country the lower the health condition of the people not from real disease but from degenerative dis-ease directly affected by those same vaccinations that are alleged to help you. Look around you and you will get the answers to these points
Countries that allow dead food (fast food) stores in, begin to see a decline in health some years later. The more of them there are allowed the more the people's health declines.
There have been many diets for people to follow, most of which do something for this situation or that situation but do nothing for the overall satisfaction of the body, the mind and the spirit.

It is so important to understand that your present state of health and energy is directly related to your thinking and the food you eat, the nutrients available for you absorb. To load up your body with toxic man-made chemicals leaves no ability for the nutrients to be taken in, even if there are some available. The little energy you get from these dead and toxic foods has to be used to endeavour to remove them and the toxins they carry so there is little, or no energy left for living.

What I am endeavouring to explain and help you understand is something very different from the normal ideas today around diets because it's about going back to basics. There are no silly fads to act out or special products that you need to buy to make this work although some added nutritional supplements and other natural products can help your recovery and continued health.

If what we have been living in is the normal then I do not want any part of it and yet the ideas expressed here should be the norm but at present, there is no profit in it for the big industry wheel and the cost of taking care of you when ill, is paid for by you in your taxes or insurance so why would they care. And Big Business own the health care model of drugs and surgery too, so they make money on all sides of your illness. Whichever way you look at it, the pain is always with you and me under the present system.

> Whether its physical, emotional or financial
> you and I are the ones paying the price
> and not getting anything in return but pain.

Now do you see why this so called normal is not really normal nor is it acceptable anymore?

> True Health comes from a place of PREVENTION
> Not POISON

And prevention certainly does not mean vaccinations.

> Think more about this and take the responsibility to take more care, consideration and respect of yourself.
> The more you take care of "YOU" NOW,

the less the cost to "YOU" in the future,
in physical, emotional and financial pain.

The concepts set out in this book is the starting point to health.
Finding out what is good for you as an individual and help bring you
to that place of prevention with the ability to repair.
The purpose of this process is to start by going back to basics, to
give your body the ability to start cleansing the toxins that you have
taken on board over the years. By going back to basics, you give
your body the chance to clear out, repair and even fix most
degenerative issues of today. Some 90% of what you face that
affects your health today is degenerative and completely caused
but the actions and controls put in place by the Shadow Controllers
to increase their power over you. The weaker you are the easier
you are to control. Your degeneration is because of they have lack
they created, the inability to thrive.
If you find you are hungry, tired or have low energy then always
drink water first then adjust what you are eating a little bit by adding
some meat, beans, nuts and seeds (i.e. protein) or perhaps more
rice, (i.e. natural carbohydrate) one or the other initially but not
together. As shown on the diamond later in the book
The reason to do one or the other at this time is to find out what
your metabolism works best on as some people for their energy
needs may lean towards protein while others may lean towards the
natural carbohydrates.
When you find the correct balance for you to maintain your energy
levels, then stick to it, adjusting only a little when needed to
maintain or increase your energy.

It is important to note here that there are no limitations on natural,
raw and fresh vegetables, so fill your boots

But remember until humanity goes back to nature to produce our
food all of it is lacking in some way or another.

Today you have been trained
To have so many things backward
Like thinking you will only be able to be happy
When you get to the destination

What about the happiness
The incredible experience
of the beautiful journey you are on
however it looks
you created it by your own choices

Talk is cheap and easy
Used unwisely has a high price to be paid
But thoughtful, considerate talk
Used wisely has incredible power
And coupled with
Action that is focus in Right intention
Used effectively brings a magical reward

3 ENLIGHTEN.

Re-tune your brain, Reshape your mind
Mindset and Intention. It all begins with you.

Remembering the quote by Einstein,

> Ignorance can be educated
> Craziness can be medicated
> But there is no cure for Stupidity

First of all, it is important to have an open mind with everything you do and especially when you read this book.
If you find yourself believing that you know something you read here as not true, do not be so quick to judge it, for when you judge you do it from a place of unhealthy arrogance of your ego. It is important to remember that arrogance is your ego acting form ignorance, from information it has made up from some past story, your own or more likely someone else's agenda that may not even be real. It is better to just observe your thoughts on the matter and do your own research. You may find that what you presently believe may not actually be the truth and it also, may not be serving you.
Your ego is a crafty character and will tell you anything to keep you where you are. Even when you are in pain, to change is a very risky thing to the ego as it no longer knows to what and where it will lead you, for it the change may be worse. There is too much uncertainty in the unknown for the ego. The ego developed for you to stay in the back of the cave where large predators could not get to you. Stay here and stay safe. This process worked for us in those early times, but the ego does not work well in modern times unless you are in danger of real physical attack. In fact, it entraps most of you into staying at the bottom of the ladder or hiding in the back of the cave in everything you do.
Therefore, you must find a way of quieting the ego. It is especially important when you find yourself rising with arrogance on or against a situation or subject. Of course, your ego will tell you, "You are Right" and not being arrogant but this arrogance and rightness

is almost always your ego spouting from ignorance to keep things as they are.

Remember you can be "Right" or you can be healthy.

As already stated above, just observe your thoughts and do your best not to judge either your thoughts or the information you receive from it.

It is also important to be relaxed about all of the following suggestions made and your attitude to where "you" are, right now. You already made those decisions so observing now will give you new prospective and information for a better future.

Make your decision to grow and expand your mind and when you do you will never return to or stay in the same dimension, emotionally, mentally or physically, it is truly liberating.

When you focus on a desired outcome, the steps needed to get there will just start coming to you for the paths to your desired results can be many.

Do not get hung up on trying to be precise, or rigidly cutting or restricting. The idea is to keep as much joy in your life as possible. If you want a treat have one now and then, just do not have them every day, as that is not a treat.

In fact, I think it is good for both the body and the mind to break from any rigidity and have a treat day now and again, after all it keeps a better balance with nature when you interrupt your normal pattern. Remember you cannot always be upbeat and positive, sometimes you have a down day and that's ok. Some say have a food cheat day once a week, or every two weeks and some once a month. Whichever you choose, do it with delight and enjoy it without guilt or worry, then go back to the better things willingly and enjoy them too. Remember to note what you eat and how it affected you throughout the week. You may find that the treat is not a treat after all as your mind may love it but your body may not.

Part of the mindset, is to decide to choose what is best for you and not to think of it as restricting or giving up in the hope of achieving, after all you will be gaining much more by feeling better both physically and mentally.

In other words, do it willingly, positively and with decisive choice followed by gratitude for feeling better.

An important note here is to understand that there are two main factors to health, the mind and the stomach. What you allow to go on in your head and what you put in your stomach directly affects the other and the state of your overall health.

I do not use the word "careful" normally as it is too restrictive and limiting, gets me wanting to become a rebel and rip my clothes off and make a mad screaming dash for the sea but this is one time it is important to be so. So be aware and careful of both the thoughts and food you put in and the speak you put out, choose wisely.

I realise that in this following section I may go over things again and again and even some what labour the point sometimes. It is for a very good reason. This section is almost always overlooked in relation to health and is probably the most important place to start as without working on your head too there is no real chance of success. The decision-making ability of your CPU depends on the right input to get the right outcome to play your music.

Having said all that there is one final point to achieving anything and everything you want in your life, and this is especially true of achieving a calm, interactive and positive mind. You must do something about it and therefore there must be some movement, some action, some effort is required to get things moving in your desired direction. This is critical.

Your Mind
I am sure as you are reading this book that you are awake enough to understand what I am about to say but If your ego rears up over this then perhaps……………………???
In present thinking it is believed, we humans use between 1% and 10% of our brain ability in a conscious way therefor this part of your mind is called the conscious mind. The rest, after the little bit you use, the 90% to 99% depending how conscious you are supposedly, is called the subconscious or unconscious mind.
In reality we use so little of our minds the we really are just about asleep so is your so-called conscious mind really all that conscious when its main function is be able to watch your unconscious actions like breathing, heartbeat and other normal but automatic functions?
In reality, most of you are functioning at a very unconscious level or more realistically are pretty much asleep

3 ENLIGHTEN.

This is obvious when you think about the fact that you only function
on much less than 10% of your mind's ability and awareness and
its more likely to be closer to around 1% or in many cases if you
look around you, possibly even less than that.

The less you use the more asleep you are and the smaller amount
of your mind you will be accessing. The less you use the more your
ego chatter pal will be talking in your head projecting pride and
prodigious. Your Ego is your very own dirtiest and nastiest little
trickster that you will ever have the pleasure to know and it will re-
frame everything, cause distraction, deception, resistance,
justification and even destabilization for you to stay as you are
when there is an opportunity or necessity for change or betterment.
It really is the devil in disguise all of your own. It does all this
because it wants to protect you from the ciber tooth at the front of
the cave you are in, hiding and safe for now in the back, to stay just
where you are.

The reason for this is that your Ego only knows what it already has
experienced in the past or even worse, thinks it knows from other
people's stories, whether true or not and has no ability what so
ever to rationalise what may or may not be about to happen now or
what may happen in the future so it endeavour's to keep you in the
past or worse, because that is all it knows.

You can see this in action, if you take a little time to look, in all the
governments, banks and big business around the world today.
There is a great need for change in many aspects of society and
the economics of almost every country but the politician's and
bankers are so unconscious they are setting up more and more
controls, deception and even causing destabilization so they can
keep you under control and keep raking in the money from us all
and not have to face the changes necessary to correct the debt
and their outrageous ideas, false or fake stories, money and debt
filled system.

Why, because you have let them have control. By doing and saying
nothing is the choice you made to accept it.

Perhaps you are so asleep you may not have even noticed it or
even worse you chose to ignore and even walk away from anything
that may have informed you because you thought it was distressing,
referred to it as negative or felt it would fog your rose tinted glasses.
It is a mistake a very big mistake to ignore these things.

3 ENLIGHTEN.

The BIG bright light of rectification will soon be at their door and smashing through it to force the change and force them out. The problem with this is that we all suffer too because in your asleep state you have been so accepting of the lies and manipulation you have been feed. You get caught up in the physical energy it produces in each stage of the process and especially in its final collapse.

If you are feeling the irritation of these words, then you too must take a good look at your ego and state of awareness.

Fear is another trait of the ego.
When a fully-grown tiger is stalking you for its next meal then fear has its function for you to get to h**l out of there quick or face being its meal. In this case it is the fear of being the meal that you will focus on and not death, which is another fear many have. It is plain crazy fearing death, as its not death itself that is to be feared but the end of life, of living that the focus is really about. So do not fear death at any point but perhaps a little fear of the end of life will help keep you going. So, Fear outside the physical is pointless as it is really just "Foolish Ego Acting as if its Real."

What about worry.
This is another cunning quirk of the ego and this time a completely pointless and debilitating quirk.
Worry is pointless self-torture based on some past misinformation or story projected on to a future situation.
The ego keeps you in it, so you are distracted from the reality of the situation. So you will stay where you are. It is only the info from the past that you can worry about even though you may be projecting it on the future. This information was only relevant for the event it was associated with and not in any way relevant to the present or future happening. It's not the same as another tiger at the entrance to your cave but it appears as if it is in your mind. When you can clear your mind of this chatter and let it be still you can ask for relevant information to help you through the present situation. Your very own mind helper has the best answers if you will only quiet the ego chatter enough to listen.
The fact is that all of the negative emotions are connected to your little ego controller in your head. The point being that the more your

ego is controlling the chatter in your head, "go to get this", "must have that", "don't do that", "what if", "its going to turn out bad if I do" and so on, the more asleep you are, simple as that. Whereas the more you can stay in a state of stillness of mind the closer you are to the awareness of your fully awakened mind where your true inspiration is to come to you.

Remember this section on how the mind works is stated as described by the Health Whispers concept. Are you confused yet?

Let's go back to how you have been led to understand it.
Your so called subconscious or really awake mind is quiet and majestic and you cannot access it when your so called conscious or in reality asleep mind with all the ego chatter is going on.

Your awake mind is self-sufficient and the symbol of guidance, the ultimate mentor. It does not get into the comparison or rating games, judgment or fault playing, or any other characteristics associated with your ego driven asleep mind. It does however put into action everything you ask for, provided it is within your life's learning and purpose.
Yes, that means everything you ask for either knowingly or unknowingly, consciously or not.
This is the secret behind the secret, the real secret to it all.
This is so important to understand this clearly, for if you ask for "want" or "wish" you will get more wanting or wishing for whatever it is you are wanting or wishing for. You will not get the results or the very thing you are wanting, you will only get more wanting it and wishing for it. If you keep saying how busy you are, more and more shit will come at you to keep you busy.

> ### This is the secret behind the "Secret",
> ### the real Secret to it all.

If you are to access you mind mentor properly you must always speak in the present tense, like "I am", "I have", "it is" "I require it to be so", "and so it is" and in the context with the intent you actually do desire it, as if you already have achieved the desired outcome, result or goal. Only then will your mind or more correctly your spirit energy take action to manifest what you are asking for.

There is also another aspect to enhance this, and that is getting the "feeling" of your being in the place of actually having whatever it is you are seeking. When you add this feeling into the mix of your seeking, it will enhance the response of your mind mentor to manifest it. There is a strange source energy inside of you, a god energy for a way to explain it, for you to create if you only ask correctly.

This can apply to everything in your life even happiness, although I believe happiness is just an illusionary perception way out there in the ether which is only drawn to you with achievement through effort and action and better called satisfaction or pleasure or joy. When you connect with your spirit energy inside then you may be able to feel happiness not otherwise available to the human singular thinking.

Being grateful for where you are right now and then require and desire to be as happy as you can be and you will be.

Your own mindset
There are five main points to this…
Thoughts, Attitude, Intention, Speak and your Actions

To start the thought process from scratch I believe mindset is the wrong word and the wrong concept for true success but again this is a big subject for another place. It is what is out there, and you may have an understanding of it so I will use it.

 Note: - There is one important point to achieving anything and everything you want in your life, and this is a calm, interactive and positive mind. You must then do something about it and therefore there has to be some movement, some action, some effort is required to get things moving in the desired direction. The desired outcome will only come when action toward it is taken by you and when movement is activated. In other words, outcome or positive mind only follows your action toward it, it does not fall out of the sky form a vision board or daily chant although every bit of effort toward it may help.

3 ENLIGHTEN.

It is important to remember that No Action is an action in itself, a choice you make not to act, conscious or not and therefore you must accept the results of this inaction. Take action, make a change of action, any action you want, if need be, do the crap you don't want to do so you can get to the place you want to get to. Start by getting up when you wake up. Decide to take action. Decide to make a difference in your life. So, in your mind decide, as force is required to get things moving then move those muscles to get up and make a difference and break your routine today that is killing you. Without movement nothing changes for the better. Yes, you can move your arm and keep stuffing crap down your neck and your size will expand for example. It may be movement for change but is that change for the better of you?
You answer that for yourself now and then review how you feel about it when you have finished reading this book.

So Note too, that the food you put in your body also changes your brain chemistry and therefore also changes your outlook and feelings just like the speak of others and your own speak does. Working on them together will give you a much better chance of success. The reality is that your brain and stomach work together and only function fully when both are in harmony and peace, this is why you must concentrate on them together.
To understand the following I need to clarify the reference to the mind. Your so-called conscious mind has daily functionality but has little influence on the world around you whereas you unconscious has infinite influence on the world around you. It will go forth and arrange things you require it to do, so that when you get there it is up to you to be awake enough to see them and action on the arrangement.
Your mind adapts and manifests whatever you feed it just like your body does. Your mind does not differentiate what it is feed it will just act on the stuff you have feed it just as your body must do with the food you feed it. Should it be negative it will bring negative and if it is positive it will bring positive into your life. What do you prefer, a load of shit going on around you or lots of good things? The choice of what you feed it is yours, however you must be prepared to accept the results it brings you. If you are not liking the results, then change the input to your mind and get a better outcome.

3 ENLIGHTEN.

The Dalai lama states

The brain you develop reflects the life you lead

I believe it should be taken one step further for clarification.
What you choose to develop in your brain is what has created and
is creating your life and reality today
 Also Remember that it took time to create what you are today, and
it will take time to create what you want to be. The amazing thing is
that it takes less time and effort to be Great when you love the
learning process, than it does to be mediocre or even average in
drudgery. The same applies with smiling compared to frowning.
DECIDE NOW TO BE GREAT.

So, the food you eat directly affects your brain and the way you
think or not as the case may be. Food has long term influence on
your brain, so the right food is key to assisting your brain to get into
the right-thinking mode. In truth they work together and support
each other. So…….

Food is not the first step, being right in the head is.

You must take responsibility for all your actions. There is no
blaming others for anything that happens in your life, especially the
condition of your health.

 Zig Zigler said it best when he said that he was almost 200 lbs (90
Kgs) overweight for many years, on purpose.
And when asked what he meant by on purpose because they said
you would not choose to be overweight would you. He said "Well, I
have never, ever accidentally eaten anything."
Therefore, it had to have been "on purpose," and my very own
responsibility, conscious or not". Yours too.

Second
Until you love yourself you will not respect yourself enough to feed
your belly the things that it loves and not those your ego mind has
construed as a way to punish your unloved self.
On the other side of your pain there is something good so hold on
to this thought every day of your life.

3 ENLIGHTEN.

You have an obligation to love yourself just as you are. You cannot change a thing of what you have done in the past which has brought you to exactly where you are today, right now, your size and shape, your thoughts and feelings and your life about you too. It is what you have created by your thoughts and actions of the past.

Today is the future of your past.

If it is not as you wish it to be, start today to love yourself and your life, enough to make it better. It may or may not be anything close to the way you would like it to be but love it just the same, as it is exactly what you have created, exactly as manifested by you. In fact, if you cannot love what you have already created how in the world will you be able to create anything better, you cannot. The lens that you view the world through is what creates the reality around you. If that reality is not as you want, get a new viewer with a different lens so you can create what you want. The lens and viewer I refer to is your mind, quieten the ego chatter and open and awaken the channel to you loving mind and interact with love. This changes the formula you put into the lens and the viewer sees a different picture. A better formula will always result in a better outcome. A better recipe makes a better stew, soup, cake.
The fact is that you are spiritually perfect just the way you are, you are not normal as normal is just average, you are not normal you are amazing, you are unique, you are a miracle, you are magnificent.
 Even if your Ego has taken you off track in the ways only such a dirty little trickster can do, you are still perfect. Until you get to be what you think you want to be, love yourself as you are right now, whatever difficulties you may have. Start with a little love for yourself at first if you have to but get started in LOVING YOU as you are right now.
Ok!
You say you want something better, well you can, although it is simple it also is not easy for most.

You can change what you want to become in the future
by changing what you think, speak and act right now, and therefore, creating a new future in you today, right now,

the better future you long for.

It is that simple but because for most of you the information you have had to work with is all mixed up and confused, it is not easy but now you have a way forward you can do it, so long as you read it all and act on everything in this book and then continue your search.
So love who you are today and what you have created, for until you do you will never be able to keep your focus on the actions you need to take to become what you want in your future creations.

It is also important to remember that what you put in your body and your mind, also affects the way you respond to everything so it is imperative that you work on both your body and your mind together so you can love yourself fully. This means thinking loving thoughts about you and showing that you love you by listening to the messages your body sends you and giving your body just what it needs.

Your Thoughts
The very first thing you must do, even if there is need for other change, is to Get our head right by realigning our thinking.

Starting again from where you are right now and look in the mirror every morning and every time you think otherwise
Say out loud to yourself, ……
"I am ok the way I am right now" and
"I love me just the way I am right now".

Put your arms out to hug that person in the mirror and as you hug yourself say…... "I love you and I am here to take care of you, protect you and feed you just the things you need to feel great."

Even though you may want to be better at something or change something in your life it is important to love yourself, as you are right now, for only then can you succeed in your betterment.

Most of the time we have our own "little person" or voice on our shoulder telling us things will be such and such or so and so if we do this or that. I call this the tormentor within. This is your very own dirty little trickster sometimes called your ego voice. Yes, that's the one that just got all defensive saying in your head "but MY ego is not like that". Don't worry just take a step back and watch and observe it and thank it for its input. As stated before everything the ego does is based on some contrived or exaggerated info of a previous experience we once had or even just heard about and then puts it into the fear of what will happen to you if you make changes to what, where and who you want to be. An unknown future even if it is assured of being better, freaks out your ego as it doesn't have any information to base what is happening or even may happen or may not even happen for that matter so it works from past information whether relevant or otherwise. See the uncertainty the ego finds itself in.

Your ego talk is always relevant to an experience in the past (or even someone else's experience) but not to this new one or any other experience now or in the future, they are each a new and unique experience and require unique responses.

Think of this and consider carefully -- would you stop talking to someone you really love, like your child, when it is clear they are not listening to you and going on doing something you think is really stupid where they may even hurt themselves. Or would you more likely keep on and on at them "torment them" to stop it. If they are important enough to you, you would keep on at them thinking you were helping them whether you are right or not.

If you really want them to listen to what you are saying would you stop and let them get on with the foolishness. No, you would keep yapping at them right. Although this is what you do and so does your ego, it is not the best approach.

You are important to your ego, it's a matter of survival.

So do not ignore your ego, do not fight it, instead you must love and protect it and only sometimes be stern with it, after all it is your own little voice so it is important to protect it like a child.

Say lovingly to your little trickster…

"I thank you for sharing those thoughts from the past but I want and trust you to help me if you can with relevant guidance for what I am doing and experiencing now, and in any case you do not need to fret as I love you and am taking care of you now".

If you repeat this each time your trickster rises up in your head and

you are having those distracting thoughts, your little voice will begin
to understand that you are taking care of it and will stop tormenting
you from the past, as it cannot help you with the unknown future so
it will stay quiet.
It is so important to pay attention and Notice and observe quietly
and without judgment everything you are thinking, saying and doing
because this reinforces your associated beliefs into you mind. Be
an objective observer and when you catch yourself thinking a dis-
empowering thought thank your chatter pal as stated above and
still the mind again. Because if you do not you will find yourself
acting it out and paying in some way down the line with, guilt, worry,
regret, frustration or pain, all the aspects of your little ego mind.
Likewise, when you are having empowering thought get on and do
them or at least something toward it right now if you can and thank
your awake brain for bringing them to your attention and helping
with the action.
When you have cuddled and protected your little voice, your ego
voice and it knows it is safe it will happily stay quiet. Only now the
really awake part of your brain can begin helping you in the present
as it has a very different set of skills and connections. The awake
part of your brain is your own very real and powerful helper and
mentor, the access to knowledge, so let it through to help you. You
will never hear its information though over the noise and constant
chatter of the ego, or if you do hear it your ego will come up with a
smoke screen so you forget it, so quieting the ego is critical.
Also, when the ego knows you are protecting it, respecting it and
taking care of it as only you can, because you are all grown up now,
it truly will stop yapping at you. Once this happens it will stay quiet
for most of the time and allow you to get every bit of relevant
information you need for any situation.
So once you achieve the quieting of the ego chatter, it is your turn
to sit up, listen very carefully and when the ego does get unruly, as
it will from time to time step back and just observe it, then thank it
again as stated above.
How about another concept to think about how this may work, the
brain is the processor of things the CPU and the real function,
manifestation and memory of everything is in every cell of your
body. Imagine that for a moment and as if that is not magical
enough, your body is filled with a god energy a spirit essence a
quantum force that interconnects every cell in awareness, like the

water in soup touches every solid so does this essence in your body. This is why your body is so often called your temple, but it is far more than that. Your brain is the inter-actor for you to direct this spirit essence. This is why it is so important what you think and speak because the power within is way beyond your present ability even to imagine.

When you get the significance of this and the ego is quiet then and only then can you have your own real, true and powerful helper on your team (the information from your spirit essence in conjunction with your really awake brain).

Your little voice the ego speak and trickster may be the little devil in your head but you have the angle right there with you in your heart.

Ask the question of it, when you get an answer, the most important aspect of this is to act on this right information, do not second guess it or let the ego go through a run of what if's about it or it will stop coming to help you. Make note of the first guidance you get and act on that and act now, do one step even if it is writing it down clearly.

Mostly you repel the success and prosperity in everything you so desire in ways you cannot consciously realise by not quieting your ego chatter and bringing your own very special helper into the place of trust and respect. It is there waiting to help and to empower you.

Now turn up your feelings of worthiness to receive and become a good receiver as it is your natural birth right as a human being to receive and not just to give.

For the story you have in your head about Not to receive, is another lie very cleverly told to you by big business because they are endlessly asking you to give, give, and give more and more to them. Stop this endless giving and start keeping and then receiving the gifts of life, love and abundance.

Note: - This is just a snip-it of the information on the power you have to manifest what you want in your life.

Tip: - The idea is to get YOU, the adult back in the driving seat while your child within is safe and being nurtured by you, and then your child within can be happy and joyous together with you.

Remember it is better to gather your own information for positive and beneficial self-brain washing than to be trapped in Societies presently sick Programming.
And the knowledge you have today and the conditions you surround it with are a hinderance to you moving ahead in the knowledge needed for tomorrow which only can come to you from you opening up to your awake brain.

> Better to be open and unconditioned.
> A nonconformist
> ## Thinking for Yourself.

Word of warning,
If you think you can use this for doing evil then think again for the spirit essence is love and does not function that way. This is all about improvement for you and those around you in positive ways.

Gratitude
This is my favourite for life and happiness. With gratitude you hold and have love. It is the most transformative of all and raises your vibration for health. Gratitude is the bringer of joy and contentment. With gratitude you can love life, love others, make better decisions and get better results. Everything is better with gratitude.
Be grateful for everything today. No matter what is happening in your life it will be better and get better when gratitude is applied. Write out at least 3 things you can be grateful for each day and more as you go along. This one thing will change the way you feel about everything for the better.

> There really is magic, in gratitude

Attitude
Attitude, or at least having the right attitude is all-important to maintain your mindset.

3 ENLIGHTEN.

Attitude is generally separated into two aspects, either positive or negative and they come from either gratitude or not in that order.
Positive is Cause and Action
while Negative is Affect and Inaction.

In life, many situations and feelings engulf us all especially in the workplace so consider the following thoughts for yourself.

Are you depressed?
or are you suppressed?
Is it a condition?
Or just a situation?
Are you controlled?
Or are you empowered?
Are you doing it by choice
Or is it by force

Now I know there are many things going on in the world today that may have you thinking that they are out of your control. The problem is that from all of our inaction and sleepwalking these things have be able to be done against us. Inaction is your consent for others to act against you, it is that simple.

Are you taking responsibility for your life so you can be in charge, in control of things in it or have you given the charge, control and responsibility to others?
This does not mean being aggressive or rude to others. You can be assertive without aggression.

Do you say to yourself when a situation arises, "how can I resolve this", "how can I do this", "what do I do to fix this"?
Or do you say, "why is this happening to me", "I can't handle this now", "I don't know how", "I don't want to"
In this context You will notice the word "how and what" when starting, creates strategies, solutions and options that open your mind to fix, repair and make good of whatever it is.
While the word "why or can't or don't or want" generally create reasons, excuses, limitations and lack that close your mind to doing anything about it. Your stuck with accepting it as it is.

3   ENLIGHTEN.

You may ask, "Are my beliefs really so important".
The answer is yes because your beliefs have incredible power over
your behaviours which affect everything else.
Your beliefs influence your inner secret source and become the
driving force behind all that you do, they affect your actions and
their outcomes in either a positive or negative way.
Your beliefs will cause you to do one of two things
Retreat and withdraw, most possibly in fear
Or proceed and act in your power, usually from a place of love.

Remember you are the ultimate salesman or saleswoman, pitching
for what you want or more likely today what you have been
conditioned to believe you can want. Whether it be to sell a car or
any other product to someone else or sell yourself the story that
you are not worthy, you are still selling. Everything you say is
selling either to someone else or to yourself and what you are
thinking is selling directly to you no matter which way you look at it.
Remember your mind doesn't differentiate good or bad thinking it
will act it out and manifest it so long as its within your agreed life
learning.
So be careful, be very careful what you SAY (or think) or it may sell
you the wrong story and therefore giving you the wrong results,
which may have you developing the wrong attitude.

What is the making of your belief system?
Remember, you were born perfect from a spiritual prospective and
the influence you have taken on from then has made all the
difference to bring you where you are right now in this physical
realm. The environment you are brought up in has a big part to play
as that will all be connected by food, family and friends.

Parents and family
When you are born your parents say to you, come on, you can do it,
just keep trying you'll get there. This happens until about the time
you started to walk and then the NOs and Don'ts begin. NO Don't
touch that you will break it, slowdown or you'll get hurt, oh be
careful you are going to fall, NO don't put that thing in the socket,
don't be silly there is no such things a fairies etc. etc. etc. this
emphasis on safety demonizes risk-taking inflicting the message of
fear on you as a child when it really belongs to your parents.

You may have noticed these are only negative statements but also very dis-empowering.
It may be better as parents to use positive statements like "Stay safe", "Notice these things and everything will be okay".
These later statements help build positive, empowering belief system and leaves you as the child with the capacity to handle whatever comes along in life.

Society and our Peers
What you see and hear around you has a huge impact on your belief system. From movies to media, the information you receive is generally negative. The thought process for example, wealthy people only think of themselves, are boring, or even wicked. They will take the money from the poor for their own gain. Generally, this is not true as most wealthy people are great givers even though they know how to control thing to get returns. There are however a few that do fit that thought process but I'm not sure they are even human as they only display reptilian traits.
On the other hand, you are told that being poor and helping others is good and that money does not buy you happiness. It is true that money does not buy you happiness but if you're poor it's hard enough to help yourself, so you can do very little to help others. Health Whispers have a saying "Be healthy, be rich and do good things for others". The key here is that you all should be doing what the very rich do and not following what they say. Even Jesus said don't follow me, follow what I do and this applies to wealth too, follow what they do.

You must look at the big picture of information to get some better grasp on reality.

First of all, the story that you are told is that you are just not good enough or you have a place to fit into society so know your place. It is under the boot of the so-called elite, right.
This story is all wrong as YOU are born a winner. Consider your Mum and Dad deciding to have you and enter into the act of creating you. With the act of pleasure, sperm is released from the male into juices in the female. There are millions of sperms and they are all on a great race against the river of juice to get to the

ovary first by swimming up the juices released in the female. The fastest and most resilient arrives and enters and that is you, the winner of the first "many millions race".

All the others are then discarded, you are the winner.

You grew and developed and eventually forced your way out into the world. You demanded to be feed and looked after. Then it was time to walk. It probably took you all, many 100s or even more times of trying to learn to walk and all the other things you learned along the way. How many of you gave up on any of these ideas and stayed crawling because it was too risky, too hard, it was too difficult or it would take far too long or even more ridiculous you were once told it was not safe to get up on your feet as you may get hurt? No, No, No. No, you persisted till you got there or none of you would be walking today.

You Are A Winner From The Start
It Is Your Natural Condition

What happened between then and now, and why do so many of you give up on the first mile, or even worse in the last meter or two of the marathons to your successes.

Believe it or not you are all brain washed and conditioned by your parents, teachers, pairs' and society. Some of what you are conditioned with is good for you to learn and some is of it is no use to you at all and some is downright bad for you.

Their intention generally is for your good, or so they would say, but remember it is their own brain washing and conditioning that you are receiving, and this does not allow you to do your own natural development.

For example, our lecturer at business school told us several times that going into business was too risky as 8 out of 10 fail. This implies failure is bad but remember learning to walk or being born in the first place.

What he did not say was that the ninth was a reasonable success and the tenth one was usually a great success. This seems like incredible odds to me when you only have to try no more than ten times for great success. Compared to conception or learning to walk this is a walk in the park on a sunny day.

3 ENLIGHTEN.

Why are so many of you focused on the negative. Why do you always get hung up and concentrate on the bad and leave off the good, positive and/or important things in your conversation.

I find it all very strange, but it may be important to remember the statement above that you are the ultimate salesman, pitching for what you want, mostly to yourself. Is it what you really want, or is it what you have been conditioned to believe you are able to attain or what they say you are capable of? Are you enslaved to your conditioning from parents, the system, bad habits or the misinformation of the bureaucrats and big business that keep you in a state of uncertainty? Is this what you really want? Please Don't let that be your reality.
 Only you can know really what is in your heart.

Your negative beliefs and self-talk are powerful saboteur's on achieving success. They will reject, repel, and push away success with such vigour that it should even be shocking to you. Until these negative beliefs are identified, discusses and then replaced with empowering beliefs and positive self-talk, not even moments of post positive thinking will help you create or maintain success in what you wish to achieve.

What makes negative beliefs so insidious and powerful is that you do not realize that you have them. For example, you may say that you want something. You may even write it down. You may even back it up with some positive thinking, but then something strange happens. You may forget names, or important dates, may procrastinate on getting something done, you may misplace something, which makes it impossible for you to do something else, you may miss an important meeting or opportunity.......... and so on. Freud said,

We are insatiable beings
and we always get our needs met.

Therefore, behind every behaviour lies a reason why things are the way they are.
You will get your needs met in a healthy way with conscious awareness or in an unhealthy way with unconscious sabotage.

Or as it is put with Health Whispers,
You will get your needs met in a healthy way with awake brain awareness or in an unhealthy way with asleep brain sabotage.

Your History
Where do we start with our history? It is said by the religious that the sins of the father are passed down four generations.
This is the consciousness connection in relation with karma.
It is not just the sins it is every little condition, happening, event especially if it had a significant impact on them. All of this comes to you through the generational line from everyone along it. The interesting thing though is that each past generation was influenced by the previous four generations and they the previous four and so on for all of your history passing on all these influences down the line. Is it any wonder you are so complicated and mixed up with all the significant events penetrating your being and all the little stuff influencing you, is in subtle ways? The whole of your history from all past generations is etched in your DNA and these are the stories the ego picks up on and reminds you of every time you want to make new things happen. Thousands of years of baggage is encapsulated in this and is dragged along with your DNA into this life which I believe is what is called your Karma, the very reason why things you do either stimulate joy or have you repaying 10+ fold. The break from this cycle is so critical for all of us and your future at this time for you are being trapped in captured energy and tradition that is affecting your thinking.
One example is being subservient to leaders, and the British anthem of the queen to rule over us is a great example. What absolute ridiculous nonsense we have all been tied into.
All the world's population have been conditioned by leaders to be subservient to them, but it is they that lead that must be subservient.
We elected them to serve us.   Look up to and respect the people that serve you the best but not just because they are in a place of influence. Remember they are your servants to serve you and us all. They are the ones that must bow to you.

It is so important today to break this cycle of past influence.

Note: We have some help with this in our wonderful universe for we are entering a new cycle where we must awaken some and there is the possibility of being able to set your Karma aside so watch out for this

Intention

Once you have your ego settled and respected your true helper will begin to help you with what you bring to it as your true intent.
What does all that mean?

No matter how discouraging your present outlook, how apparently unpromising your future, cling to your desire and you will realise it. Picture the ideal conditions, visualize the success, which you long to attain; imagine yourself already in the position you are ambitious to reach, and then release it. Now do not acknowledge limitations, do not allow any other suggestion to lodge in your mind other than the success you long for, the conditions you aspire to. Picture your desires as actually realized and hold fast to your vision with all the tenacity you can muster until something better is manifest This is the way out of your difficulties; this is the way to open the door ahead of you to the place you want to reach, to better health, to looking and feeling great, to better and brighter conditions in every aspect of your life. Applying this to everything will bring you success in achieving whatever it is you want or can dream of. Holding the final desire in mind will show you the steps needed to get there and remember one small step or change today may not seem like much on the day you do it but keep doing these small steps and changes makes a huge difference in the years to come.

> It is not just what goes on in your mind,
> It's what goes out to the either
> And into your body that counts
> As this affects what happens outwardly
> And within.

This statement applies to all life, all situations, all eating but especially important to what goes in your head because your head is the director of your operations, the guiding hand of what you do, say, feel, how you act, your attitudes and what you eat. It is the

3 ENLIGHTEN.

master of where and who you are at present, of everything you want, of all that you have achieved to date and therefore also that which you will do and achieve in the future.

1st it is a must to work out, know, picture and then desire what it is that you actually want to do, have, become or dream of.
If you know what you want great if not you will have to start from where you are and what you don't want then get all you don't want written down, everything, think of as many reasons as you can try to get to 100 to start but keep going if you have more. And add at the bottom of the list "All of these things I do not want in my life and any more I think of along the way, will no longer be part of, connected to, or affect me again from this point forward. My mind is focused on better things." Now read this as you burn it at the bottom of your garden. The act of burning is only recommended here at the beginning to magnify your intent. Intent is the key here.

So the next step is to actually work out what you do want so you can desire it. Start on the list of what you do want as you did above and do your best to get 100 or more. Don't worry to much about putting them in order as they will change as you receive.
Then pick out the few that you feel must happen soon and start with the most important.
Your whole thought current must be set in the direction of your desired goal. Live in the conviction that you are progressing, advancing toward that which you want.
Note: -
"You will remain a victim of your situation
As long as you have only that vision."
Or
"You will become a success of your situation
when you change and have that vision"

Your mental attitude, your heart's desire, is your perpetual prayer, which interestingly, Nature always answers.
Do you realize that your desires are your perpetual prayers — not head prayers to an outside force, but heart prayers to your inner spirit and that they are always granted. Therefore pray wisely.

3 ENLIGHTEN.

There is a tremendous power in the habit of expectancy, of believing that you shall realise your ambition; that your dreams will come true.

Note: The laws of nature may not allow your desire to manifest if it is against the natural law. In other words, do not use this power against others for retribution or personal empowerment over them as nature may reject such an outcome or even have you paying a huge price for your actions. This works for positive empowerment that helps you and everyone around you.

So, I repeat – know and be clear about what you really want and that it will help everyone you connect with.

Some examples on Speak

It is so important to ask in the right way.
For example, a friend is always saying he needs more money.
Most of the time he goes out and finds a penny or two on the street and wow now he has more money. Now I do believe it is important to pick up those pennies when you are gifted them as it shows the universe you respect and value what it can give you but in his case he was just getting more money.
Anther friend always tells me how busy they are, and I ask why would you say that because you will just get more shit dumped at your feet to do and that is what she says always happens to her.

Have you ever been to the restaurant with a woman who puts her handbag down when she sits at the table saying, "I must not forget this when we leave"?
When you all leave, she leaves without the bag. The focus is on the word "forget" as the mind does not understand "must not".
To remember it, it would be better to Say, "I must remember it."
The mind will attach to the word "remember" and you will remember.

You are always trying to lose weight but are always putting on the weight. The focus is on the word weight, so you put on weight.

3 ENLIGHTEN.

Changing what you say really is empowering so Say something like "I am slim and healthy"

We are our best and worst salesman or woman so say only what you really want, understand this because what you say in all instances, really does become your intention. It is so important to understand this.

Helpful Tips

You can post a real picture on the fridge or wall of a person, situation, place that you want to aspire to be like, have or be. It can be physically, financially, fame or however you yourself want to be, like or have. By doing this it will help you to keep the mental picture you have of your goal alive. You must spend a few moments each day in focused thought toward that goal. The more you do this the more power you unleash within and the faster the results. Remember if you are not there yet you have not yet put enough in to receive it.

Set out your thoughts and ideas about what you really want to achieve and write them out as goals in the present tense as if you have already achieved them. If you can get to 100 positive reasons for doing it and 100 negatives' if it doesn't happen then you will have power behind the desire. This may even take some weeks to become clear of what you really want. Do not worry if your goals keep changing initially. You will eventually get there.

1. Start and end every day with a few minutes quietly thinking about your goals and visualize you have actually achieved them and do your best to generate the feeling that it would give you.
2. Feed your mind with positive ideas and thought (rejecting any negative thoughts and ideas)
3. Review your plans for accomplishing your goals daily and adjust as necessary.
4. Think of better easier ways to achieve what you desire.
5. Reflect on all the valuable lessons of your life and apply that which will help you toward your goals and a better life.

6. No matter what happens temporally today that may seem like a setback or holdup stay focused on the goals you want to achieve.

Speak, and Changing the words, you speak.

What you say is very powerful not just in your life but also to everyone around you.
Think and say only that which you wish to become true and never speak with intention to harm others as it may also harm yourself.

Thought: -
To start with, let's get this out of the way. You may say you do not like salespeople calling and bothering you all the time but remember almost everything is selling. You are selling to others what you want of them and even more importantly you are selling to yourself with everything you think and speak every second of every day so saying you don't like sales people is the same as saying you do not like yourself. Your ego chatters away at you with all sorts of random stuff. The problem is that your mind does not know or care about the difference between positive or negative speak of anything you say, it makes it happen, good or bad you created it. So, love salespeople as you can learn a lot about yourself from them.
A friend always used to say a throw away comment at the end of the day from time to time that went like this. "Another day older and deeper in debt". He began to wonder why he could not get ahead financially, when I explained the power of his words to his own mind he has since changed and is seeing the benefits. The power of your words on your life truly is significant.
Therefore, say and project only the positive you really want for yourself and those around you. If you do not, your mind will get for you that which you speak of even if it is not what you really want but you said it anyway. It brings you what you speak of.
A friend was thinking of summer and commented how it was great when she was "fit" as they say and could wear a bikini on the beach. Now she is so self-conscious she won't even go to the beach let alone wear the bikini. When asked she says "she worries

about what she looks like, her weight and wishes the beach was only imaginary and was no longer to go to. A swim in the sea is defiantly out because if friends of the earth were about, she would be rescued from the shallows and towed out to deep water. No more pictures on social media to be critiqued and so on.
Nothing in her anxiety and self-loathing helps her loose the excess as it catapults her to the nearest sugar laden comfort. Exercise is out because you know what those at the gym will say and anyway there is no gym wear, she can fit into now." She is fat shaming herself all the time while saying the body image she wants is unattainable and anyway it is normal today to be fat and all those films and adds are abnormal and more.
All this negative speak, limits any possibility of improvement of body let alone life, stop it. It's true that about 60% of you out there today carry way too much fat and you are growing fast in size and number. Yes, there is every size and shape imaginable, as many as the number of people but the key here is, is your size and shape today the size and shape for your optimum health. If it is you are one in twenty four, lucky you but read on to keep it that way as I am a lucky one too but it got me in a few short years no matter what I did to stop it, to 20 stone and I wasn't even talking the wrong talk..
Always remember that you choose this life with the parents you have so you are most probably as near perfect as you can be when you are born, it is what goes on in your head and that which comes from the heads of others around you that upsets the true balance of life from then.

Start by understanding
your words are your thoughts in motion,
your mind puts into action this motion
and creates whatever you project,
so be aware, very aware of this.

Look in the mirror and Say out loud to yourself "I will no longer speak with forked tongue to myself or anyone else, with lies or negatives, to manipulate. I now take full responsibility for using only positive and loving speak in everything I say"
To repeat ……
Think and say only that which you wish to become true and believe with all your heart that you will do as you have just agreed to

yourself to do whenever you say everything. For example you may say you hate salesmen or being sold to but remember you are your own greatest salesman or saleswoman as you sell to yourself every time you think and speak even if it is your little ego self-talk and irrational chatter, it all gets manifest.
Again, I say be ware

Here are some words that I recommend you remove from your vocabulary when talking about food in the context of the present-day information.
They are "weight loss", "Diet" and "low fat" and some others generally but that is a further subject.

And some of those reasons why, to think about

"Diet"
The first three letters should give you a clue and the last letter indicates today i.e. DIE-Today. Stop right now with all dieting and no longer DIE in the diet. Dieting is like playing Russian roulette with your health. Diets are killing all possibility of you achieving the thing you want most "weight loss" by just depriving you of the food you want (or more probably need) most. More importantly it's possible that why you stop losing the weight after the first week or so may be because you are only losing some water content when you diet, the very thing you need to buffer your cells from the toxins, to remove those toxins and repair your body while you are still loading the body up with toxins from the diet foods .
After all what does the word losing mean? Trailing and Failing.
The diet industry fuels false promises with 100 million plus people on diets each year, that fail and then most add extra weight on after they finish dieting. Failed dieting brings unimaginable profits to the diet industry as the people go back again and again after the false promise of losing weight while blaming themselves for their failure and not the useless produces, they are taking. I believe it will be seen as a criminal act in the future to make money from the pain and failure of others.
Even Daniel Abraham the Slimfast producer says he has helped millions of people pursue their dream of being slim, but never does he mentioned anything about anybody actually achieving that goal for the long term.

3 ENLIGHTEN.

Weigh in at weight watchers or any other weight loss group and chase the dream of being slim. It's just that, a dream and the reality of how to achieve that slimness is nowhere to be found there. It would be better to buy a lottery ticket as you have more chance of winning than losing weight and keeping it off with such programs. All the problems you have before you start will increase with dieting Dieting is psychological and physical torture, a complete con and can cause serious health issues, in some cases even death. I recommend not putting yourself through it for any reason on this beautiful earth.
If you are on any sort of fad diet then stop it right now as it is slowly killing you and your wallet, adjust to a more balanced thought process.

All extremes are forms of imbalance.

The diet industry is making billions on the back of the your failure to achieve weight loss. If dieting really worked, they would not have a business for long. It is such good business that all diet products are now being made within the food industry. Its money for old rope with constant return custom for them.
All degenerative dis-ease's, obesity and neurological issues are Chronic conditions caused by the dead food epidemic of today. Dieting food is even more dead and gives you even less of everything than even normal food.
Replace this word diet with; food, meal, breakfast, lunch, dinner, chocolate, anything but the word diet in any context of dieting to lose weight.
Do you get the picture yet?

"Low fat"
It is most unfortunate that we have been misguided in this way. The scientists may have had some compelling reasons (which I explain later) for it in the beginning but the information was never thought through or researched fully otherwise we have been scammed again.

If you do absolutely no exercise, then Animal Fats may need to be reduced, but not those from plants or fish.

There is a consideration however, of what is called fat, and here, consider Good fats as referring to all things natural (without any act of pre-processing or heat treating). In other words, all natural produce with no more processing than the following – cold pressing, stirring or mixing gently or in some cases home cooking, for example all natural plant fats like avocados and cold pressed olive oil are great provided you do not heat them.

Animal fats, fish and eggs are great fats and do not change with heating the way plant fats do

This means that all other fats, for example., polyunsaturated and trans fats, I.e. -all Veg oils whatever they are called, margarine's and all things made with these trans fats are out and should not be used at all.

While cold pressed oils and all natural fats like olive oil, butter, animal fat, lard, can and should be used in your food regime.

Low fat and diet food and drink
is actually helping you to put on fat

Low fat and diet food and drink is actually helping those of you that eat them, to put on the fat, as your body is tricked into thinking it is getting food benefit, only to find nothing, it screams out to you for more and you supply it with the same empty process. Over and over again, you are being tricked into doing this until you reach the half-ton man or woman. The other concern about low fat and diet food and drink is the complete lack of any nutritious value at all so your body become malnourished, weak and sick. You may think you are ok, but the strain is there. It has built up over time so you fail to notice the change but if it had been instant (like getting the flue) you would know you were sick and seek and search until you found help or better still do something about it yourself.

If FAT really was the problem,
then the Eskimos would be long dead.

Just remove these low-fat words completely from your thinking and speak and even more important from your food.

"Weight loss"
If you are over size then reducing your size is a very worthwhile

thing to do for your long-term health and wellbeing at whatever age you may be.

The first consideration however is to understand the meaning and effect of losing weight. Muscle has weight and is significantly heavier than fat. Are you really considering reducing your muscle mass? I think not, so stop wanting to lose weight.

All the excess you have on your body is made up of fat and toxins which is relatively light compared to muscle, size for size. It's just that some of you have so much of it that it weighs heavy in comparison to the rest of your normal body mass. It is also important to note that as you go down the fat road into sickness you will have a lot of water retention too. Now this is heavy to carry around and is such a relief when gone.

The importance of this understanding still applies, and you would be much better to use the correct speak.

What you must aim to lose, is Millimetres, Centimetres, or Inches. In other words, measurement. The measurements to be considered is not height but around the waist, Butt, Legs, Arms, Neck.

To be in excellent condition for example, the waist, measurement ideally should be 50% or less, of your height for men and a bit less for woman. This will depend on your Individual body makeup of course and is just an estimate. Therefore, the height need only be considered when you are considering your ideal size around the belly. Then again you will know you are on the way to good health because you will no longer be feeling heavy, blobby or blur, but lighter, more balanced, good and even great. A feeling of being well or even liberation.

It is also important to remember that exercise builds muscle and therefore also adds weight. This of course is defeating your attempts to lose weight even though you may be healthier than you were before you started. As you can see here the goal to lose weight is a false goal and unachievable, while to lose measurement around yourself is a far better aim.

"I Can't"

Never say "I Can't" as they are some of the most self-limiting words you can ever say. Even though you may think you are saying them to someone else, it is yourself in truth that receives the message and your mind then rejects and dismisses all possibility of doing anything related to what you say these words about

"I Don't know"
When you say, "I don't know" you will always draw a blank as to "how to". Think of taking a road trip to visit a friend and you say I don't know how to get there you will find you have no ability to find a way to actually get there. If you say it in a different way like "I will need to ask someone, search on the internet or look on a map to find my way" then you have your mind opened to find a route to your destination. The same applies to anything you want to achieve, like losing weight, being healthy, finding a new job or income source or even finding a new girlfriend or boyfriend.

"I know"
Ah yes, I know, a favourite term of the moment.
 When you say "I know" your mind knows there is no need to even think any more about the subject as you already know all there is to know. Again, this will shut out all possibility of moving forward on the quest in question.
Just like in the journey above if you say "I know" your mind thinks you already know so there is no need to find out how, what or why. This will kill your possibilities just like "I can't" and "I Don't know". This is another way for your egos to stop you in your tracks and hold you just where you are, eliminating all possibility and the energy to achieve it.

"Label yourself"
This does not seem so important as everything is labelled in our world, but the money changers know the power of labels so have manipulated things this way. When you label yourself with anything that is not helpful to you it will hinder you as your mind takes on the meaning behind the label. e.g. If the doc says you are diabetic, and you accept this and say "I am diabetic" your mind will create such an outcome no matter how hard you try to do something different. Even the simple words "I think I'm getting a cold" will ensure you get the cold for you have already accepted it in. When you take on and accept a label you then have to accept that result. It is far better to just thank your ego thoughts, your friends or the doc for

their opinion and defy the outcome by demanding and expecting a different and better outcome and therefore result.
It may take a little time and yes it does work

"What if"
What if is a destroyer of everything great. It is the egos trickery to distract you so you will not remember anything good and stay just where you are. Unless it is used in a positive suggestive way, avoid it
Watch closely your thoughts and words to change your thoughts for a better outcome.

Enlightenment - tips.
Remember your words are expansive and immensely powerful results generators so use your speak carefully and only in the way you wish to create and manifest your goals in your life.
The following is to help you (and to remind you) to take responsibility, ownership and control of your speak, your mind, your body and then your life.
Freedom is only possible with some structure to support it and not as Janis Joplin sang when there is nothing left to lose

Using the acronym of the word "control" as a base to build the support structure for your freedom to develop.

CONTROL

C - stands for clarity.
Be clear on what you want (and not what you do not want) for whatever you focus on is what you get.
O - stands for obstacles.
Whatever is in your way to what you really want then to sidestep it, find a way around or over it. With this action you will find the obstacle much smaller than you had 1st imagined.
N - stands for now.
Now means do whatever is necessary or even whatever can be done, right now, to take you one more step closer to what you really want.

3 ENLIGHTEN.

T - stands for tipping point. What can I do right now to tip the balance, solve the problem, find a solution to move on?
R - stands for responsibility.
How can I be responsible, become the course and take action?
O - stands for opportunity.
What, where and how can I learn from this and grow?
L - stands for leverage.
How can I leverage my learning's and actions above?

Habits to establish today for success:
1. Declare and align with your successes
2. Understand resistance and when it does or does not benefit
3. Create a support system for your new habits
4. Move yourself forward
5. Expand your compassion (for yourself and others)
6. Assess your progress (it's not the ways you may think of! Do not compare with others but from review to review of your own assessment of your personal progress)
7. Powerfully visualize what you truly want (once you have worked out what it is)
8. Act courageously (even when you feel afraid)
9. Take inspired action steps (there IS a difference!)
10. Understand that gratitude catapults you closer to your goals
11. Align your energy with the things you want more of
12. Understand and accept that some setbacks and failures are actually beneficial
13. Make valuable adjustments while on your path
14. Understand that giving actually puts you in the right place to begin receiving

Above all else – Fill your life with as much joy as you can and be happy for any reason.

"Being happier doesn't have to be a long-term ambition. You can start right now. tackle as many of the following as possible. Not only will these tasks themselves increase your happiness, but the mere fact that you've achieved some goals today will boost your mood.

3 ENLIGHTEN.

1. Raise your activity level to pump up your energy.
2. Take a walk outside. Natural light and the colours of nature stimulate brain chemicals that improve mood. For an extra boost, get your sunlight first thing in the morning and feel the benefits all day.
3. Get a nagging task done. Crossing an irksome chore off your to-do list will give you a rush of elation.
4. Turn off the mad screaming mis-informers, the MSM news, that fills your head with negative fearful nonsense and inform yourself from citizen journalists telling what's really happening in the world. Our world is filled with incredibly negative speak today, from news to neighbours, change yours by informing yourself to think for yourself and speak a better speak with love for yourself and those around you.
5. Create a more serene environment. Outer order contributes to inner peace, inner peace demands outer order and a place to decipher the information. Truth or not.
6. Reach out. Having close bonds with other people is one of the most important keys to happiness.
7. Do a good deed. Do good to feel good—it really works!
8. Learn something new as often as you can.
9. Always Act happy.   Don't Fake it, feel it. Decide to be happy. Some people worry that wanting to be happier is a selfish goal, but in fact, research shows that happier people are more sociable, likeable, healthy, and productive and they're more inclined to help other people. By working to boost your own happiness, you're inspiring other people to be happier, too. You see, YOU being Happier, is also benefiting others and that can hardly be selfish.
10. Every day write a list of 5 things every day you are grateful for that day. And make your own Notes on your Happiness and how you are feeling today and do it every day: - the more positive you are the happier you will be, and this will also improve your health.

The purpose of this chapter is to help you to understand where you are today, to help you learn to start loving yourself.
It is important to remember that your little ego voice function's only from its memory of the past, it uses reason and logic to get your

attention to agree and hide in safety but your real power of function is to create that beautiful velvet silence within and connect to your own internal mentor where you can live in synchronicity.

When you love yourself, you will respect and treat your very own temple, your body, the way it desires to be treated. You will listen very carefully to the messages and feel the feelings it sends you to feed it only the food that supports it and brings it love. Until you do, what you do with the ongoing information will be more difficult to maintain, sustain and therefore get the real benefit from.

One final tip:
As your little voice cannot help you with the unknown ask it to remind you to have fun, to laugh and dance, to feel the joy in your life. It can do this because it remembers the essence of the joy of life while young even if you don't feel them now. Living in joy is the first great step to everything human and especially your health

LIVE in JOY,
The first great step
To everything Human
In health and everything else
Be as happy as you can be for any reason
Love yourself for every reason
For you are a beautiful spirit.

4 INSPIRE.

Removing the Offender's
Should the modern medical model be on trial

> Sometimes it is better to Kill the perpetrator's
> before the perpetrator's kill you

The problem regarding health and disease today is that about 98% to 99% of all health issues of today are dis-ease while the other 1 or 2% is actual disease. What this means when explained is that 2% or less of the issues you face today you are infected with actual intruders of one sort or another that you must defend against or correct their balance inside. The rest of the health issues of today you are not being infected but affected.
You are affected by pollution, artificial chemicals, dead food, nutrient deficiency, GMO's, stress, social conditioning, bad thinking and of course your own sleep walking belief that what you are told is true and so, so much more. Mostly it is what you put in that is causing you to be affected in the way you are today.
Another way to put this, is it infectious disease, infected or degenerative dis-ease, affected.

Where do you begin?

There is nothing in the modern medical model that has the ability to show how this works or even show a difference when you follow this information here or not but you will feel significantly better over time and that has to be a better way to live, in a place of feeling better. There is also in the development, equipment that can show more of how things work and help enhance the body healing process by stimulating the nervous system and so on but they are at present not accepted within the medical model because they would show you how to be healthy and there is no profit in you actually being healthy.

If you are not working, living and eating to enhance your health and prevent problems you are in reality choosing to accept the results of the terrible yet unnecessary degenerative dis-eases in your life. Everything health comes from first living in unity with nature and this means having a healthy digestive system. Your stomach is the central organ for a reason, and everything stems out from it. When your gut is unhappy there is a pass on effect. You will feel the pain somewhere in your body and brain. When your stomach is happy so too is your body and brain.

> ## Removing the offenders
> ## Removes the inflammation within

So why did I start with being right in the head? The main reason for the last chapter is, until you have the right attitude and love for yourself you will not love yourself enough to do the things necessary to help and heal yourself. You will not feel you are worth it, if you have any self-loathing and not love for yourself, why would you take care of the beautiful you and the amazing body you were born with. If you need more love for you than you can give yourself then seek help, come join our community, ask for a hug, do something because you truly are worth it. When you understand the complexity and yet simplicity of nature that you are, your very existence is truly a miracle. Treat yourself as one with tender loving care.

Make it a priority to find the love inside for yourself and your inner child for without it there is no real chance of health or anything else. Now that you love yourself let's talk more about health.

The Offenders.

A young friend Michael had developed allergic reactions to different things on different days. He never knew when it will strike, what was causing it and to what severity he would suffer. The problem is that when he finds out about one thing that's affecting him and cuts it out, then another thing would strike. He has also tried eating the alleged offender again and had no reaction.

It was all very strange and the Doctors had no answers to offer him other than endeavouring to put various labels on it and prescribing more and more toxins i.e. drugs in the hope of disguising it so it would appear to him that the doc had done something.

Unfortunately, there are more and more of these stories showing up all around the world today that did not exist at all even a few years ago let alone100 years ago and yet we are told health is better now. Yea right a cow may one day jump over the moon too! We went through the process set out in this book with the extreme act of removal of the offenders below and his known offenders also. This was completely trial and error I have to say, as was his Doctors approach to him, but this time without any more added contamination of doctors Drugs to his system it was certainly worth the effort as nothing else tried had any shown real benefit. To date he is doing better and has less reactive strikes than previous and he says it is amazing how much better he is generally, just by removing the foods that he found were affecting him. There is still a way for him to go as of writing this to get fully healthy again even though everyday there is progress. To see him now is amazing compared to how he was but when you get so compromised it does affect how you feel about the setbacks you will all have in cycle of progress Remember it takes time to heal the inside. The key here is that he had been to many doctors and they could not see that his diet was what was causing his issues.

> ## Doctors just want to label it so they can poison it.

His belly was so compromised and out of balance that he has to push down on and starve out the bad bacteria overgrowth which fight hard, before his own good bacteria can build and grow. His condition has also allowed toxins into his system which have stressed the cells and this can sometimes take month to settle and may only do so when the stressed cells die off and a new cycle develops.

While in the UK recently I read of a lady who has an agonizing allergy. Despite tests and hospital visits, doctors have been unable to diagnose the problem. She states it's like a mixture of the worst hangover and being poisoned. She is absolutely right. This is clearly and exactly what it is, "being poisoned" by the very foods that are supposed to support her and then drugs added on top.

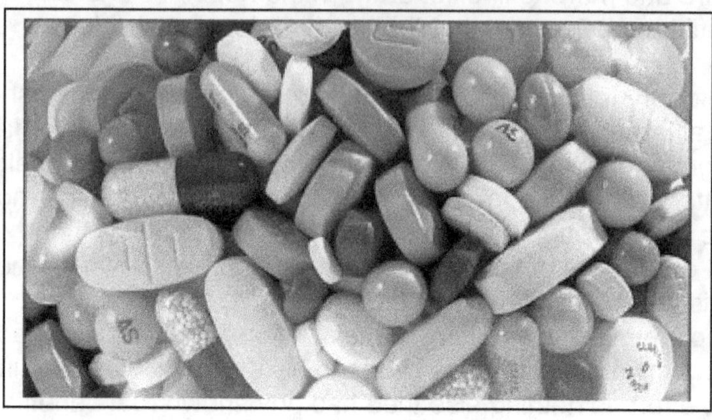

Unfortunately, as said earlier
Doctors just want to label it so they can poison it.
It is pure madness, trying to fix an already compromised self
with even more toxic sustenance's.
Are you all MAD, yes one would think so by what you do today.

Having said that it is important to understand that there is a place
for the doctors and even sometimes their drugs where you have a
condition that at this time requires the drug to maintain your system
or reduce the pain some. Although pain is there for you to do
something about it so killing pain totally is not always such a good
thing.
The modern medical model works great in the first stage of it, the
diagnostics but then it all goes wrong with the labelling followed by
treatment by drugs or knife. The problem I see is first the label they
put on you and then the drug they use to disguise it. The Label
because it gets into you mind and you own it as if it is real which is
not a good place to be because it is not real. The disguise is not
such a bad thing for a short time, a month or two till you can do
something to actually understand the cause and then start the
repair which they never do, so this disguise goes on for years and
then the direct affects (which strangely are called side effects) from
these are causing so many other and sometimes very serious
issues, which need disguising by even more drugs, again and
again. Another no-good situation all the while the original cause
has not even been looked at. This is today's medical model and if

drugs don't work or disguise it enough, they want to hack into you to have a look around, called exploratory surgery. The insanity of this is like a science fiction horror story on steroids.

Modern day life is filled with artificial chemicals from industry, farming, food processing and from the medical model itself, these chemicals affect you in ways that bring unimaginable physical and mental health issues. they cause imbalances of all sorts even to make men effeminate and woman aggressive. While all the dead foods the chemicals and toxins just stay and build up in your body. Never having the ability to be removed because you have no real live un-compromised foods and truly natural water to remove them. This is what you must work on, however you do it, removing the intake of the offender, whatever it is, is the key and next step to real health.

As stated earlier what you put in your body directly affects your minds and your thinking, your responses to everything around you and especially how you feel about yourself, what you have created within and without along with others. You will also see when you take action how it improves your body so your memory will also improve and there is a very good reason for this effect as told in a later chapter. Understanding this should give you more incentive to work on your mind thoughts, your speak and your body. When focusing on just one, it is more difficult to achieve what you want without the others being considered and included.

Healthy body and healthy mind will also bring you to a better place to create a healthy family with healthy finances which then develops a much healthier society around you.

The process – what you MUST take out

What most of you eat and drink to keep you going or in the hope of an energy boost may give you a small increase for a short while, maybe 15 to 45 minutes, then an energy crash and the need for another shot. That is what it really is, a shot, as your body is really running on empty, plus your body is having to work hard to deal with all the toxins in most of those so called foods and energy drinks that you shoot at it. It is even worse than that though because most of the foods available today in the western world are chemical laced from the methods of production, processing and even packaging. These chemicals are designed to kill bugs, bacteria and fungus outside of you but when you eat those same foods the same effect is played out on all of your own microbes that you have inside you that are absolutely necessary for you to thrive. Those little guys, your Microbiome inside you for your natural daily function are killed by these chemicals and dead food and your gut is compromised. Continue this and the bacteria you do not want come out of hiding and thrive and grow out of control and your gut becomes eaten up and the layer of good bacteria that protects and filters the food you eat for absorption is gone. No barrier of protection of your gut means all the wrong stuff gets through into you blood. As it flows around your system it compromises every cell it contacts especially your brain. Your defenders kick into action to remove these toxic bodies foreign to it and because the inflow is constant, from all the chemical laced food, they too get traumatised and overwhelmed with the task and cannot switch off until they die themselves. This means that when you compromise your gut with chemical toxin's and dead foods it takes three or more months of no compromised foods to stop this cycle of trauma and therefore for you to start to feel better. The longer the compromise of your gut the longer the repair cycle. I have seen some recover in a few months, but others take a year or more. The problem here though is that when you break the cycle in the early stages of repair and eat compromised food again your gut is again flipped back into the compromised state and the repair cycle often has to start all over again. Do not break your good work of repair at the whim of some candy crush or sugar rush.

If you find you are hungry, tired or have low energy, remember that it is not coffee or energy drink that you need but the right food to replenish your energy. What most of you eat and drink to increase our energy may give you a small artificial boost for maybe an hour but after that there is a crash. Then you need another shot. All the while your body is running on empty.

Importance of Removing the Offender's
Starting from the point that your Gut and Digestive system is the centre point to your health then it stands to reason that this must be the focus of your attention when thinking health. If you are not supporting the little helpers in your gut with the things, they need to thrive then you are killing them. When you kill your helpers, the harmer's take over and cause havoc in there. Without the

protective helper layer everything gets through, into your blood and then your troubles start.

All your physical, mental and emotional wellbeing
is generated within and arises from your gut.

When your gut is compromised by intolerance your body stress levels are increased which affect your body's ability to respond. Keep stressing your body with bad foods and reducing it's ability to respond and eventually you end in a health crisis and suffering.

Sometimes it can take years for issues to manifest themselves as ill health and sometimes there may be no way back as the scars of your abuse of yourself are so hardened. Do not wait to be ill get on with loving your gut the way you must.
It is important for you to eat only the amounts and the types of foods your body responds to best. There is no one size fits all for we all have unique body needs.
None of the offenders are doing you any good. In fact, the invisible pounding your body and organs get from consuming these offenders is tremendous. Instead of removing these offenders most of you wait until you get sick or just do not feel well, so you head to the doctor for some magical cure all pills.

Unfortunately, the remedy you get from your doctor, whatever they decide to prescribe, has an 80% plus statistic of actually making you much worse than you were before you went there.

Using yet another poison (proscription drugs) in the idea of fixing your body after years of eating offender foods (also poisoning you) is the crazy idea of modern medicine, in reality its insanity as stated several times in this book. I will go on stating it too because it is just that, insanity.

The lies you have been told to believe
are so the pharmaceutical and food industries
can keep on prospering at your expense.

> Think, for who does the story they tell, benefit
> and you will see it is not you.

Now as said earlier there is a case for your Doc and their proscribed toxins from time to time and in certain situations, but there is no justification at all for it on every situation and all of the time as is done today.

The must Removals review.
First things first – Refined Sugars of all types, Artificial sweeteners, sugar, fructose, sucrose, corn syrup, aspartame and any other you come across whatever they are named.
Before we start on this let's clarify that sugar is just another form of carbohydrate, in an extremely refined form and there are about 50 plus names for all the contrived forms of it so be aware, inform yourself and remove them all.

- Collect all items containing your processed sugar and artificial sweeteners
- Check all items for any other type of refined sugars in the content
- All processed foods and drinks even breads, cookies, and cakes.
- Put all items with sugar products in them together under lock and key so you cannot use them or discard completely

Note! If you will not discard these items, use them very sparingly over the next few months or so. Watch closely and feel what your body tells you when you do eat them.
Use the Health Whispers Food diamond for a better guide to eating. Research all the products you are buying and Stop buying any with the above from this day forward.
Note! This applies as well to fast foods like burgers, fries, taco's, sandwiches, chips or crisps cookies, sugar pop etc.
Note! If you must buy these products then only use them very sparing, but we recommend not buying them at all especially in the first 6 months so you are not tempted to consume them and by then you will not want them if you have done things as suggested here.

Vegetable Oils of all types:

All vegetable type oils that are being palmed off on you whatever they are called you must avoid if you want great health and you don't want to spend the last years as an invalid from a heart attach or Stroke.   From veg oil to palm oil, canola to corn oil.

The following is the original use and should remain so

- Canola oil, used both domestically and industrially and in fuel industry as bio-fuel.

- Cottonseed oil, used only as industrially.

- Palm oil, used only to make biofuel. The worst of oils because it not only kills you it also kills the orangutan.

- Peanut oil (Ground nut oil), a clear oil.

- Rapeseed oil, including Canola oil, for external use only

- Safflower oil, until the 1960s used in the paint industry.

- Sesame oil, for external use only

- Soybean oil, produced as a by-product of processing soy meal and for external use only.

- Sunflower oil, commonly used to make biodiesel.

- Olive oil, used in cosmetics, soaps, and as a fuel for traditional oil lamps.

- An exception possibly, is when and only when they are cold pressed to remain in their original form from the plant but all of the processing of today does not leave them in their natural state. The only one we have found that does is olive oil when cold pressed correctly.

All of the above to be used for external use only unless you know they are fresh and cold pressed. There are many more oils and names of oils around the world important for you to avoid and never ingest.

This subject is very close to me as I have lost several friends from this with grave suffering, so I have done extensive searching on the health-related effects of these oils on us all. I have to say that I get so angry with the advertising lies and misinformation of today, especially about these products. As I write this book another close friend who did not heed the advice and continued using vegetable oil for all cooking methods suffered a massive heart attack with all arteries fully blocked. Solid with sticky congealed vegetable oil deposits. No blood flow means the heart stops and no heart beating means no oxygen to the brain or any other organ. Very quickly starting with the brain everything deteriorates and dies. Strangely doctors now consider this normal but still have no consideration of what possibly could be causing these sticky deposits in us although it is implied it is cholesterol.

Another thought to consider is that these oils may not clog your arteries if you are vaping for example, but it will clog your lungs, block your oxygen intake and create an environment for real dis-ease to start. If you value your health do not consume them in any form.

All heat-treated oils are for external use only.

Now there is the consideration you must understand of what is called fat and what is not. This must be considered now as you have all been told that all fats are bad except veg oils and produce made from veg oils, i.e. low-fat spreads, margarine's etc.
In fact, it is just the opposite that is true as these vegetable oil products are just shutting your system down and blocking the ability of your body to work as it is intended to.
All natural produce (animal fat's like lard and butter) and others like cold pressed olive oil or natural produce in its original plant form that has a high fat content, like nuts, coconuts and avocado's, are a must to be in your eating program provided they are as nature made and produced them.
That means produce, with no more processing than the following – cold pressing, stirring or mixing gently. In other words -- All things natural (without any act of pre- or high-speed processing or heat treating) are in fact very important to include in your eating program. As stated earlier there is an exception to the heating and processing as Animal fats are great for your health and can be heated by cooking without problems.

To clarify, this means for e.g., polyunsaturated and trans fats, i.e. - veg oils, by whatever name they come up with to call them and there are many, margarine's and any products containing these, processed into artificial oils/fats are out and should not be used or ingested at all, while cold pressed and natural fats, oils like olive oil (provided you do not heat it), butter and lard can and should be your choice to eat.

Now you may be thinking that vegetable oil is a natural product and yet I have just called it artificial. Yes, the original oil from the vegetable may be natural but the extraction and processing process changes it so much it is little better than an artificially produced substance.

It is very interesting to note that doctors often comment on the build-up of fatty deposits in the arteries of people.

They say cholesterol is the problem when there is, good stuff and bad stuff, too much, it sticks to the arteries. This is caused by too much acid in your system and as a protection method the cholesterol creates a layer. When you look more closely you will see it is the vegetable oils sticky residue is creating the layer that is blocking all the receptor sites and arteries and that is why the cholesterol rises as there is no way the body can use it for benefit so it just stays and circulates.

Strangely this is now more often also put down to eating the fatty foods from animals. It is also interesting to note that when you look at the waste from any of the foods you eat, they have a fatty appearance unless of course you are just eating grass or hay. It may be prudent to add that even the sewers in modern cities today have huge problems with sticky fat blocking them that did not happen so much before the low fat and vegetable oil fiasco.

Also, if you go back prior to 1970 people ate much more natural fatty food, were usually slim and most did not suffer with the problems we do today. Could this mean that the build-up of fatty deposits in the arteries is not caused by you eating natures fat food but actually caused by eating vegetable oils which stick onto your arteries walls stopping any of the natural systems of the body from working. Is this the real reason that you have high blood pressure and high cholesterol and lots of other bad stuff just floating around in your blood stream, because your body's ability to work is blocked by a sticky gooey hardening vegetable oil stuck on the inside of your arteries, veins and all over your cells. Is this the reason you are heading for a heart attack and stroke in the near future like every other person around you?

You bet your life it is.

A great experiment for you to do. Take a moment to put a small amount of vegetable oil in a small shallow container.

If you have not done this before, do it now. Leave the container on the windowsill for a while. It may take a few hours to several days depending how deep the layer of oil is, for it to thicken to a sticky substance. This is exactly what happens inside your arteries, veins and all over your cells. You are the reactor effect to harden this product just like plastic is hardened but this time it is inside you as a sticky layer.

Yes, this is the substance that is causing the so-called plaque build-up your doctor says is caused by fat or cholesterol. Yes, it may be true that fat is the cause, but that fat is all the various types of vegetable oils and their associated products, and not the animal fats implied by the present misinformation.

Your doctor tells you to have only vegetable oil and no other fats. Remember, there is no money in the truth for the medical industry and your doctor, even with their initial desire to help are also being misinformed about this stuff by the drug salesman.

Wheat

Today's wheat products and sugars
are the cause of the Obesity epidemic
and a major factor in all degenerate dis-ease.

This may seem like a bold statement to make but you only have to look at the graphs of sugar consumption increase overlaid on the obesity and degenerative health issues graphs and it is clear evidence that they are the cause and wheat now too for reasons I will explain. The same may apply to barley, rye and other grains. Collect all your items made of/ from or with a wheat content and discard and please do not buy any more.

Today Wheat Flour is just another sugar as it tricks the body into thinking it has eaten something of value, only to find there is nothing but sugars to assimilate and waste to dispose of. Your body can not do anything with this sugar other than use a small amount of it for energy and the rest is stored as fat and toxins most probably to get it out of your body as soon as possible and/or put it into a safe store just like your computer does with the bad stuff. The waste that is left is another problem as is rots and ferments and sticks around and creates a beautiful heaven and food supply for bad bacteria to explode and over run your good guy supporters. Neither safe nor satisfactory for good health. As soon as this process is done, your body comes back to you asking for more, as no food value was received. Unfortunately, you eat the same type of dead food and the cycle continues over and over again. Obesity followed by sickness will sneak up on you along with all the other problems and dis-ease associated with this type of eating.

We may all think that wheat in itself, is a great product. In ancient Roman times for example, Egyptian wheat was a main staple of the Roman armies. Even in the United Kingdom during the early 1900's it was considered one of their most healthy times when there was a huge consumption of whole wheat products. Note the word whole as in, complete. So yes, it was a great product, until production was changed after ww2 by intensive farming with artificial fertilizer, added chemicals, modern mechanised processing and regulation was introduced. Then throughout the following years a manipulated version has been developed with short thick stems so the loss to weather was less and therefore the production more, in this manipulation process the structure of the grain changed to having very little nutritional value but the gluten levels increased. Today's wheat is a little more than a foot tall but when I was a kid it was about three to four feet tall. Unfortunately, today it is not a great product because of the manipulated structure, production methods and the processing it goes through before you get it. This leaves the product dead and without even the minerals you need to digest and assimilate it let alone get any benefit. Basically, all that is left are sugars and waste. Have some cake with your coffee as a treat now and again if you really must, yes, but do not eat any wheat-based products produced in the west, in large amounts.
If you do not think you have issues with gluten intolerance then you may be deluding yourself, make a change anyway as a crisis for you is nearby. At least try a better wheat-based product like

couscous or bulgur wheat. Although I do not believe it is just gluten that you may be intolerant to but other aspects within wheat itself or even more likely the lack of the necessary nutrients to allow you to process it. Apart from sugar the rest of it is waste so what can your body do with it? In the process of trying to remove it, it has attracted mass bad bacteria to feast on it and eventually take over your gut destroying your own delicate gut balance. No natural gut balance and your internal food processor is weakened and then stopped, and you lose the ability to absorb the fuel you need to function. Turn off the engine and the car stops. Not only do you feel tired and fatigued through this process, the acidity builds throughout your body with joints starting with pain and all the way to the big C. When you add this dead waste on top of the sticky vegetable oil deposits throughout your body you are in for a disaster and dis-ease is not sneaking up on you it is rushing at you like a tsunami to crashing over you. From muscle and joint pain to gut and bowel issues to plaque blockage and heart attack or breakaway and stroke, and you will say "I didn't see that coming". Before that you may have killed off your good stomach supporters which form the protective layer to process out the things not good for you and allow into your body those that are. The good little microbes of bacteria, often called by the few doctors that are interested enough to learn about them, your microbiome that you depend on, because there is nothing for them to feed on and process for your digestive absorption. Instead you feed the bad microbes with this rotting mess of waste which not only gets everything inside your gut out of balance it goes on to fully destroy the protective layer and your filter is gone allowing in everything, toxins and all to have open door access to flood your body with harm and pain. Is it any wonder you feel bad when you eat?

Until wheat is produced in a natural way with all the nutrients in nature, as is needed and used to be, for the plant to bring in the minerals for you to be able to digest it, do not consume and compromise you gut with it.

Dairy
Consider carefully your consumption of dairy. Health Whispers recommend you not drinking milk at all. In the natural world only

infants drink milk and that is from their own mothers.   Never do they drink from another species under normal development. Other products made from milk are in truth no better unless perhaps those made from unprocessed sheep or goats' milk. This is because of a different enzyme that we have as humans been consuming (sheep and goats milk), in its unprocessed form, for many thousands of years and the body has developed some ways to process them in the gut provided they are in their natural state. This is not the same today due to the Heat treatment or pasteurizing required in today's regulation riddled and restrictive society.

Further consider that Cow's milk is a relatively recent introduction to the human diet and has different enzymes to that of sheep and goats, and the human body finds it very difficult to process even in its natural unprocessed form. This is even more difficult with the modern-day processing that is required in this very regulated world. To add to this problem the processing kills most of the enzymes, the very thing you need to help you process the milk and what you are left with is really just a toxic whey substance. To top this off you choose the low-fat version, the only bit that may have had something for you to gain from the milk, the fat is gone and what is left is just waste. The waste that is left leaves your body struggling to know what on earth to do with it. In reality this waste just creates a fermenting and rotting substance for your bad bacteria to feast on increasing the takeover of your gut and system.

For those that consume milk and wheat together, when you pour this milk over the rotting bed of flour just imagine the happy in house feasting party your internal destructive bad guys must be in.

Low fat and diet food and drink
Low fat and diet food and drink actually helps you to put on the fat, as your body is tricked into thinking it is getting food, only to find nothing of value, it screams out to you for more and you supply it with the same empty promise. Over and over again. You can be tricked into doing this until you reach the half-ton man or woman. The concern about low fat and diet food and drink is not just the empty waste along with the complete lack of any nutritious value but also adding insult to injury with the massive amounts of added salt and sugar, so your body not only gains fat but also becomes

malnourished, weak and sick. You may think you are ok, but the strain is in there. It has built up over time so you may fail initially to notice the change and its effect on you.

If it had been instant, like getting ill, you would know you were sick and seek and search until you found help to put it right.

Unfortunately, when you are so secretly compromised with low-fat and diet food and drinks you have no such possibility of awareness until its almost too late.

If you are even slightly overweight, you are directly affected by this and most probably have a degree of addiction to fast and/or processed foods and diet drinks.

The more obese you are the more the addiction and therefor the bigger the intolerance and the faster the time bomb of ill health will explode within you. Stop it now.

Other things to consider

Orange Juice

has no nutritional value. Unless the oranges are picked fresh and ripe and squeezed straight from the tree the day you drink it there is little chance of any value. Also the longer it is the more the acid without the C will affect you adversely.

Starving yourself

Although I recommend reducing your food intake or even do a green and water cleanse from time to time, never calorie count ever or starve yourself on an ongoing basis. Your body is getting little enough goodness from the food you eat today as it is, without that. When food is fully natural and nutrient rich then fasting may be of benefit but food does not come close to this today.

Eat right, Don't die-t.

Soy

although a good product in its natural form it's not worth eating today as most of the soy in the western world is produced in the USA. Genetically modified and processed to hell leaving almost no value in the end produce and leaves your own immune system in compromise along the way. To add insult to this, veg oil is often added to bulk up soy.

Salt
Like everything in relation to food all salt is not equal either. The everyday table salt has many additives and generally is bleached out of existence so has little benefit for your body. This is also what is in all processed foods in very large amounts which is bad for you. So much so that if you had the same proportion in just water it would make you sick.

Wherever possible only eat fresh and natural food that you prepare yourself and only use sea or rock salt from a reputable source to taste once it has been cooked. If the food is of nature and not chemically produced it will have taste itself and does not need masses of salt in the cooking of it.

Note
Those of you that live in America will struggle to find chemically uncontaminated, natural or non GMO foods unless you grow it yourself, which strangely some states are passing laws to prevent the concept of home grown sufficiency and collection of water. These are your basic rights, but the present-day controllers are out of control over greed and power and there seems to be plenty of sleepwalkers ready to enforce the controller's stupidity against humanity.
This book is mostly about food and its effects on us but there are many other offenders that you would also be wise to be aware of and if possible, remove.

Remember: everything affects you wherever it comes from
Intake is not just what you put in your mouth,
it's what you breath and what you put on our skin
and is also what you allow into your head
and that which comes out your mouth.

You are all exposed every day to foods with little nutrition, laced with manmade chemicals from artificial fertilizers, herbicides and pesticides, hormone and antibiotic filled meat. A myriad of chemicals in every product you buy, to petroleum and other toxic chemical filled skin care. You all live and drive under a rubbish layer of dirt, dust and chemical filled air, especially when you live in a city. The bigger the city the thicker the rubbish layer.

For example, Soaps, Cosmetics, hair and skin products and deodorizers.

There is little that can be said that will stop woman and some men from applying makeup because of the ill-conceived pressures of society that you must disguise your natural beauty with a mask of make up so this is going to be very brief.

Consider what is in the products that you use. Remember your skin is your largest organ and whatever is laid on it will be absorbed into it. The areas of skin most exposed with substances applied to, are the hands and face, unfortunately for you they absorb far more than other parts of your body so even more reason to be careful what goes on. Just like your gut, when exposed to other factors your skin becomes more porous and allows more to pass through to the inside.

It is best to take care of the skin from the inside as described in this book and assist the protection of it only with natural products on the outside.

This is an extreme case but hopefully you will get the idea. I once knew a heavy machinery mechanic who for about 20 years had washed his hands and forearms with petroleum products and especially brake fluid to get the grease off when he had finished his work. He suddenly felt ill starting from his hands and forearms being very heavy and was soon unable to get around as his muscles became stiff and very sore and very quickly ceased up altogether. They just did not seem to work anymore. This kept getting worse and worse until one day he was virtually paralyzed and needed to be helped to do everything. Within a few months he died with a doctor's report of natural causes. The natural causes were that his body had no longer been able to tolerate what he had been doing to it and he really died from a slow build up into toxic shock, once upon a time called polio.

Yes, this may be an extreme case but every one of you are putting these petroleum products and other toxic chemicals on your skin. They are in almost everything now a days.

Note:

4 INSPIRE.

When you break the cycle of the early repair period and eat compromised food again your gut repair cycle seems to go back to zero and you may have to start all over again.

RESEARCH FIND AND USE
ALL-NATURAL PRODUCTS ONLY,
FOR YOU AND YOUR FAMILIES OWN GOOD.

Watch out for marketing gimmicks that entice you into wanting a product. If they have to trick you into wanting it, its most probably a lie that its good for you.

All of the above mentioned invade your body by stealth, slowly building up to a crescendo of dis-ease that is unhappiness for your gut. What comes from your gut unhappiness is any condition you have from skin problems, muscle and joint pain, cloudy eyes, grinding of teeth, especially at night, to brain fog and depression and many more compromising your gut. Why? Because everything gets out of balance with these products mentioned above and your supporter microbes get overtaken and can no longer protect, filter and support you. If continued this will cause more issues which compound your compromise. The wrong food produces the perfect environment within your gut and intestines for an overabundance of all the wrong microbes and a feeding frenzy environment for all sorts of parasites, large and small. We all have them, however in the natural healthy state they are under control by your own supporters but when your supporters are pushed aside or die off from starvation your health goes downhill fast. Close your eyes and wait for the crash.

If it's been a lifetime of dead food then removing it is a great first step, but you may need to do more to repair your microbe balance, mend your gut and get rid of the parasites. Until you do, true health will avoid you.

Taking the Impact to inspire Further
These next few realities you must also consider.

Fizzy Pop

All the fizzy pop companies are the largest buyers of sugar and plastic. These are two of the most toxic and polluting products on the planet and they take no responsibility for the results of either, your health or the resulting plastic pollution, although you strangely and foolishly chose to participate in their crimes against you and the planet.

Coca-Cola for example is the biggest producer of plastic bottles on the planet (millions sold every hour) but do nothing to fix the problem of pollution from their production of plastic bottles. If you stopped buying their toxic drinks there would be no waste to fix and it's not just them, they're all doing it.

Milk and its production

It started in America in the pursuit of higher profits, like so many things it has spread through the industrialised world. Production of milk in some parts is now in the extreme of intensive farming. This is where a small Farm of about 25 acres or less has a smaller fenced off area where the cows are kept, a hundred or so in each small fenced area. They never leave this small area unless they are sick or are going for a trip to the slaughterhouse when too old to produce milk. Their fate is to eat hay and meal, to lie in mountains of their own shit, are pumped full of antibiotics and other chemicals in an effort kill the disease that festers in their udders in such conditions and be milked twice a day 365 days a year. Their only exercise is to walk around the small pen and going into milking. Their only respite from producing milk is a few days, sometimes, when birthing the next generation of cow slave.

Note:

This small pen process also applies to beef and chicken producing farms today.

This is just the first problem with the milk of today. For many thousands of years humans have kept small animals and have therefore had the use of a small amount of sheep and goats' milk. This was always fresh and eaten daily or made into a soft curd or cheeses to be consumed within a day or so. Sheep and goats milk also has an enzyme in it that humans have developed the ability, over time, to digest.

Some 90% of cows however as an enzyme in their milk that we cannot digest. This enzyme issue may not be such a problem when modern processing is considered as all that is left is a lifeless waste produce anyway.

The next problem arises when the milk is taken from the animals living in such poor conditions, full of disease, it is trucked and mixed and processed and heat treated to such a degree there is little, or no value left. The only real value it has to you, the fat and that is usually in is taken out and used elsewhere due to your low fat fiasco, the enzymes destroyed to such an extent that you have no chance of digesting it and what is left for you is about as much good to you as airplane toilet water. Some of it even has a similar colour so it is whitened with paint colouring to make it that rich white colour you think is the colour of milk. In nature most things have a very slight yellowing to them.

Now do you still want to continue drinking it?? I certainly don't.

Hamburgers

Interesting statement from McDonald's as they say their burgers are healthier than most other hamburger and fast food joints now, because they now have up to 5% meat in their burgers. Yet, they have always advertised them as 100% beef.

Therefore, what is in them if it's not meat, yet 100% beef?

Well are you ready?

Yes, it is probably true that it is almost 100% beef.

When all of the meat and cuts that are possible to sell elsewhere are taken off to package to sell, the rest (i.e. waste that was once only considered fit for animals or fertiliser) is dumped together into a big machine to be stripped, mushed and mixed till it comes out in a big slimy pinkish mess. Because it is stripped and mixed with bone, offal and all of the sinew and fats and scrapings from the bones and skin, it is subject to contain any diseases that the animal carried. To kill any possible disease contamination this slim is soaked in vats of ammonia and possibly other household chemicals. Next, it is mixed with the binder and preservatives, as this pink slime (as it is actually called) will not stick together. It is coloured (and McDonald's say they add some meat) and made into those dead patties that you stick between those lifeless air buns. Great food, right??? No wonder it gives most people a headache. So Why did they expand this process of feeding it to humans?

Firstly, why waste good meat that you can sell for profit elsewhere on something like a ground up mess burger when you can get a similar look from the waste with a bit of creativity.

Then you may remember some years ago there was a thing spreading the Western world called mad cow disease. It became clear that what was causing this was the dead animal and waste products all ground-up and fed back to the same animals. At that time, dead and diseased animals were added into the mix. No problem right, just feed it back to them.

There was no requirement considered to use anything like ammonia to kill off disease that may have been in this waste because it was only used as animal protein.

Thought: We are at the end of the food chain and we all know, if you have been awake the result of this mad experiment on the humans affected by this horrendous practice.

Because the waste carcasses of all animals were ground-up together, disease spread across the animal species, one example is from sheep (scrappy) to cattle (mad cow).

As you may know, cows, sheep and goats are not meant to eat themselves. They have evolved and developed to eat grass and other vegetation just like rabbits.

When this cross contamination came to light in mad cow disease the process was said to be discontinued.

Therefore, they say to themselves "What to do with all the animal waste. Ah, let's change the process a little and feed all of it to humans." Although we are told it is a different practice used, it is the same in principle with just the mechanical mix and fix that is different. And recently we have been told that there may even be human remains all mixed up with this slime, it's a long and sad story how the dark controllers get rid of the evidence of their crimes, and you may have turned cannibal without even knowing it.

Now you can see why Fast food Burgers taste the same all over the world. Eat these pink slim Burgers at the fast food joints at your peril.

This is sad but true. This is yet another waste and disposal issue resolved by human consumption like so many in today's world.

Incidentally America claimed that it never had any Mad Cow Disease, while the rest of the world struggle ed with it. Yet the practice of feeding their own Blood and Bone back to the animals as it was called started there. Although they do not have so many sheep to pass over scrappy, the feeding of beef to themselves also cross contaminates. We had many reports of its existence there, especially in those small caged farms even though it was and still is denied.

We are no longer convinced that this practice is not still continuing in some way or another in some places.

Aluminium pots and Alzheimer's

It has been stated for years that aluminium is considered a contributing factor in Alzheimer's and aluminium pots are the main cause. But are aluminium pots really the cause or even a contributing factor to Alzheimer's.

I have seen people all over the third world that use aluminium pots daily and some clean them with handfuls of sand too because of their primitive conditions. They have done so for years but they do not suffer the same cognitive conditions suggested to be caused by these pots.

Is it really the pots we use in our homes, or could it be something used in the system allegedly for your benefit and to distract you from the truth you are told to look at the pots, as it always is, it must be your fault, right?

Could it be the aluminium sulphate put in your water supply to make it look crystal clear as described in this book. Perhaps also other chemicals found in the water and food supply, beauty and appearance regimes could also be considered to be contributors. For example, in almost every underarm deodorants there is an aluminium additive to block sweat. You happily put this on the glands under your arms close to the blood stream carrying the chemical directly to your brain. It is all very easy to distract the people from the truth and put the onus back on all of you while industry and official practices continue their misinformation for profits.

Also if you are awake even a little you will have noticed? What about the spray that is added to the aeroplanes and dumped high in the sky, nick named Chem Trails These are not part of an aeroplanes normal output which is a Contrail, or condensation trail. Contrail's are "streaks of condensed water vapor created in the air by an airplane or rocket at high altitude from the hot exhaust emission and only last for a very short distance behind the plane until cooled again by the air and evaporate. Just like your warm breath on a cold winters morning. When you do finally see these chem trails for what they are you will be in a place of disbelief in the official line of disinformation.

The Chem trails
are a very different story from Contrails, for they are chemicals added to a separate system in the aeroplanes to spray the world and especially over cities. Why you may ask, then you will have to ask the Shadow controllers for a true reason but I can only think it is to toxify the earth so you will have to buy the seed made by Monsanto as your seeds will not grow and to toxify you so you will die early from dementia. Already I am finding that seeds are harder and harder to get started even though some years ago there was no problem.
There have been many independent tests done over the past five to ten years and not one of them are good. It has been confirmed that all around the western world especially, a cocktail of dangerous and extremely poisonous chemicals are being dispersed. This includes aluminium, strontium, barium, cadmium, nickel, mould spores, yellow fungal mycotoxins, and the best — radioactive thorium. This is not the total list. The one chemical that is being sprayed the most is aluminium. It can cause all sorts of health problems. These chemicals and especially aluminium primarily attacks the central nervous system and can cause everything from disturbed sleep, nervousness, memory loss, headaches and emotional instability. It especially shuts down the nervous system killing the connectivity of your processor to your memory store throughout your body. Since the increase of this mad chem trail spraying has intensified over the last 25 years or so the increase of dementia has increased some 20 times and is now the number 1 cause of death, wait for it, in the so called civilised first world. These practices are not civilised and nor is anything else they are doing that you seem to be asleep to.... Nor will it be, so long as we have Shadow controllers having their way that you are asleep to. Wake up to this and withdraw the consent you have given even if it was unknowingly
Now I hear you say again that I lose you when I say such things but it is you that are in the losing position for until you realise,

understand and acknowledge that these things are actually happening you and all of us cannot correct the wrongs against us. So please at least keep an open mind and check it out for yourself. And watch out for their conspiracy angles for they are strong on this subject as they have much to hide and deny. You will know the conspiracy is against you and me if they call it a conspiracy theory.

Reconsider everything around you and especially the use of all products with nonsolid aluminium additives.

Organics:
Organics today are not what we believe them to be although still much better than intensively produced foods.
Again, the American government through the FDA and lobbying from the FDA's partners in the food and chemical industries of America forced a change of the rules to allow some spraying of chemicals on organic produce.
Once again, the Shadow controller's dependable's in the US government, doing the industries bidding, have forced these rules on the rest of the world so that America can sell their chemical contaminated waste into world markets without restriction.
Yes, organic produce may be better than intensively farmed produce because there should be no artificial fertilizers used but may still carry the residues of other deadly sprays along the growth cycle. This also depends on the commitment of the farmer to the meaning of nature and organic food so find your local grower and ask.
Truly Intriguing would you say?

Thoughts and tips
Imagine your house filling with gas. The gas rises slowly and unnoticed, soon it is almost up around your waist so you can still breath ok as you walk around, and you don't really notice the problem developing. You feel that something is not quite right, and you may even sense an odd smell you cannot place but you think it must be all right as there is no obvious issues you can see. It is time for a break from your daily chores, so you go to the kitchen to make coffee. As you turn the machine on there is the smallest unseen spark inside, and boom, half of your house is destroyed.

There is a similar effect inside your body. The offending products causing your irritation, builds and scratches at its chosen location until the spark effect triggers some major degenerative issue.
This section is about your gut and no longer loading it with bad and toxic foods that create sensitivity and intolerance and preparing to feed it right. Strange how when you look at the shape of your gut it looks a little like your brain only bigger. There is no coincidence here as your gut and brain work together. Hence the reason I have started it this way in this book. Feed your gut right as it calms and enlightens and stimulates your brain in the positive. Create the right story in your brain and you will only feed your gut with the supporters that take care of both. The two are so closely connected, I believe they are one. They are both processors, like duel chips in your computer doing different jobs to support you as a whole. The slight difference is that when your gut is off everything is off even eventually your brain.

One final note on intolerance
When you eat something that you are intolerant to, it may not show up immediately, especially in the early stages of intolerance, or you may not get the reaction immediately. It can be a few hours to several weeks before the full impact or reaction is felt. This is very confusing for most as your mind does not work this way, but it is in fact how things go. The only way to prove what it is, is to keep a diary to see the lag time of reaction from what you eat, drink or even that which you speak, which can take even longer to manifest.

Wheat products are a classic example of this in the early stages of your intolerance to it.
A friend has these issues with irritable bowl. Every time he eats wheat, especially bread or pastry, he has a lag of several days so refuses to relate it to these so called foods yet believes his issue with dairy as that is same day affect. Even though he is fine when he stays off them. Some of you are slow to catch on but you must be observant to start with and intuitive too to finally get and understand the messages your body sends.

5 REGENERATE

Introduce your Supporters, The healing process

The right food is your best medicine
Although you can do much healing with the right mind input, it is important to combine this with Food as it is the best medicine of all for your body, or more correctly the right food for you is your best medicine.

> When you feel the reaction
> especially in your gut,
> take action to put it right.

And the joy of a happy stomach

> When your Stomach is happy you will be happy
> feed it correctly
> as it will bring you a happy brain too

There are a few other things to consider regarding your supporters. When I refer to protein I usually refer to meat and you feel put out, please just rethink it as a good quality vegetable protein of your choice.
The point is, you must have protein for full body and brain function and I am not suggesting overriding your free will to choose what you eat for this protein as that is not for me to do, it is for you to make your own decisions on these things.
Remember that is not just what you put IN but also what you put ON that is important.

Note:
You have seen this applied above to the mind, now let's apply it to the body. This will support what you are doing with your mind, your thoughts, your attitude, your happiness and the decisions you take into action.

5 REGENERATE

Introducing Your Supporter's

The best place to start with anything in life is to first educate yourself and this book is an introduction to your education. It is also important to take it further and do your own research. You will find the truth is out there even though sometimes well-hidden in the shadows on purpose. You may wish to start by proving what is said in this book and that is a good start, however there is so much more to discover when you look further.

Sleep

Sleep is the most overlooked and underestimated aspect to health and a clear mind. In today's fast-paced world most of you don't get enough sleep. This seems like a ridiculous oxymoron when you have so many time-saving devices at your fingertips however more devices that save time mean that you can do more and therefore fit far more into each day. This is because you are busy doing all of the extra time-saving stuff your time-saving equipment allows, requires and others expect of you.

What has the lack of sleep got to do with your health and/or weight you may ask. Well a lot in reality, because when you are sleep deprived you tend to eat more and want it now, if not sooner. Junk food is the quick and easy fix for you and even more so when tired. And more importantly when you get into a deep sleep on a regular pattern your body system kicks in repair mode to fix, repair and replace your cells as needed. Without this deep sleep cycle, it may only be able to do a half ass job if at all so you forgo the necessary updates.

It is therefore imperative to know how much sleep you need in the cycle for repair and do everything you can to make sure you get it, for the lack of it is extremely detrimental. When you are in a deep sleep you recharge the circuitry throughout the body and brain for the next day's activity, and concentration.

Sleep is most important for dealing with stress or grief, for repair and healing your body, the balance of your own chemical and hormone makeup and even more importantly set in motion the removal of unwanted toxins. The clean-up and repair process is so energy intensive that it is not possible to do it while you are awake, especially the clearing of the toxins from within the deep tissue and the brain.

Don't get enough quality sleep and these toxins will just stay there and build up and eventually be the cause of numerous dis-eases both in disorders of the nervous system (neurological) and other physical dis-eases.

Why is sleep so important
your brain can only be awake and aware
or in sleep and repair
as there is not enough energy available
to be both aware and repair at the same time.

Considering you cannot help but consume so many toxic foods and generate so many by-products from them in today's world, that must be removed while you are asleep. For good health this is further indications of the importance of good sleep.
Some research shows that the best time of the night for chemical re-balancing and repair is when you're in your deepest sleep somewhere between 1 and 5 in the morning and that you need to have been asleep for approximately 4 hours before the peak time for the best results and benefit.
The peak time therefore is somewhere between 2 and 4 in the morning so therefore it is recommended that you close your eyes for sleep by about 10 PM. Now this may not be possible for those of you working shift work but whatever your normal time for sleep, set out those parameters so you can create in your own sleep cycle to get to the peak period at a similar time each day.
It is also considered that most people need some 8 or 9 hours sleep every night which even I find difficult to achieve in the present time of expectations on us all.
To take it one step further, sleep and good water are most important for great health, getting the best from your food, to balance your own chemistry, to boost your energy levels and help the body to function without the stress from food or life.
Something else to consider here is that it must be natural sleep and not sleeping pill induced. They may shut the brain down enough for you to think you are sleeping but the cleansing and repair process does not take place. There are also very severe affects from most sleeping pills and that is around 50% plus increase risk of loss of concentration and memory loss leading to possible Dementia and Alzheimer's over time.

If you decide you have to take them for some reason or another then as with all Pharmaceutical's, never take them unless necessary and never for more than two or three months at a stretch. Get your adjustment in as quick as possible to resolve the issue so you no longer require them.

Again, if you need sleeping pills to sleep you will most probably be suffering an intolerance to some kind. If you have done the effort on your thoughts and self-love effectively then food or combination of foods and or drink is the next best place to start to find out what may be irritating your body to disturb your sleep.

Another consideration in todays world is all the devices you are addicted to, computers, tablets, phones and so on. I have found that when used at night before sleep you will take much longer to actually fall into a deep sleep. This is because the light they emit has the affect of early morning light on your brain, time to wake up. This is the last thing you want if you need a repairing deep sleep. What to do then is to get your addiction out of the way earlier and commit to putting them away at least two hrs before it is time to sleep and do not look at them till the morning. This will help with settling your brain on all sorts of things too as now you are in control. Try it and you will be amazed at how much better you feel and sleep through the night.

Remove these and provided you drink plenty of good water you will soon find yourself sleeping through the night. Check out the section on intolerance too. Like all things nature it may not happen in a day it may take time.

Some sleep tips
1. Be grateful and thankful for who, what and where you are right now.
2. Drink plenty of water throughout the day and a large glass of water before bed and take another one with for night supping.
3. Stick to a routine for bedtime and wake up time.
4. Avoid using phones, tablets, computers or other led and/or back lit devices for an hour or two before bed as their bluish light tricks you into thinking it is time to wake up.
5. Avoid long catnaps in the daytime.
6. Eat your main meals at breakfast and lunch and lighter in the evening and never just before bed.

Laughter

The great healer. This is totally overlooked in relation to health and possibly even more important to health than sleep. Find something to laugh about every day if you can. Laughter seems to naturalise the bad chemicals you have in your body that are there from stress and bad eating, fear and the ego-based activities. Laughter also sends shockwaves and pulses of energy through your system disrupting the standard or compromised state and bringing in ripples of repair and healing. Just like a stone into a still pond these ripples spread throughout your entire body to create an amazing healing process. Laugh a little and a lot whenever you can. Watch a funny movie or read a funny book, have some fun with a friend and if you cannot find anything to laugh at just stand and laugh at yourself, go through the physical motions of laughing out loud starting with a hahaha, hahaha, hahaha. Even this will change your state for the better by the vibration waves sent through your body. Your little child ego voice cannot help you with the future but if it feels safe with your love and protection it can help you to feel that childhood joy and laugher again, encourage it to bring joy and laughter into your life at every possible opportunity

Whatever it takes laugh, laugh and laugh loudly.

Water:

Drink at least 2 litres of pure good quality water each day. You may need much more than that as some may need up to 5 litres and if you are in a hot climate you may need even more. Your body will show you how much is needed in the way you are feeling i.e. clarity (clear head) flexible and smooth muscle action and skin and feeling of well-being.

Note: This is over and above any alcohol, soda, coffee, as these have other problems and work for the body to do and filter. Some are also diuretics or have extra salt and/or sugar so further reduce the water content available to your body.

Who needs Botox when water does a far better job?

Water even keeps your brain from shrinking (along with proper nutrition) especially as you get older and, in some cases, when the brain shrinks it can lead to increased memory loss. Not because your memory is in your brain but because of reduced brain function and connectivity to your body system .

If at all possible, find yourself a quality water filtration system for your home or office that not only filters for pathogens and chemical contamination and toxins but also find a means to add back in the mineral content and life that has long gone.

The world is now saturated with chemical toxins that have leached into the water supplies and rivers from farms, gardens, homes, and excreted and discarded pharma drugs.

Tap water may be safe to drink from bacteria but the treatment chemicals put in to kill the bacteria, are not even filtered out or removed, nor are all the extra chemicals from agriculture, rural and domestic applications, that have found their way into the supply. Even worse are the residues of all the prescribed, prescription drugs given out by doctors. Some only have as little as 10 or 20% absorption into the body (and just as well or they may even kill the taker they are so toxic) while the rest is passed through and ends up back in the water supply. Remember the water is continuously recycled in most cities so there is no escaping all the prescription drugs in the water. There is a deadly cocktail of all these toxic chemicals and drugs in all your water supplies so special filtration is needed if tap water is being used.

Therefore, it is not advisable to drink straight tap water because of the possible toxin levels from garden, farm and industrial chemicals to heavy metals and waste residues and the Doctor's prescription drugs. Even in small doses these can build up to excessive levels that your body cannot handle in the long term.

Also, if you live in any big city it is likely that the water you are drinking has passed through many other people before you. In London and New York, it is said to be about 11 to 13 people that will have drunk it first, then you get your chance.

The human body is said to be approximately 70% water by mass and 90% water in the cells, so it is not an exaggeration to state that water intake is most vital. It is possible for you to live for 30 days and more without food but survival without water is at best 3 to 5 days. Even 10% loss of water can be fatal. And water acts as a natural cooling system, provides protective cushion for tissue and is essential for digestion. Water helps remove the waste, carries all the toxins out of the body, giving space for it to carry the nutrients and oxygen back in to replenish and nourish your cells.

Good clean and fully mineral enriched water is essential for all aspects of good health. In most big cities today, there is no mineral content in the water so you either find a way to reinstall them or you need to take supplements because they are not in the food either.

Spend some time out in nature
Following on from sleep and water, is the importance of being out in nature, do some gardening, go bare foot in the park, lay on the ground, do some staring at the trees, you may even see them watching you too and sending you love, soak up the beauty of nature, walk and lay on the bare earth and receive its magnetic standing wave energy, fill your eyes with the light of the day, receive the gifts of nature. This includes the sun for it brings you the gifts of life. As we are light beings will we find in the future that the sun can sustain us in every way? From it's so called vitamin D to the full range of light in colour, frequency and energy.
I do believe there is so much for us to learn about the sun, the beautiful ray in the sky the true giver of life.
All are necessary for your wellbeing; nature works as a whole so you must get all of it to be truly healthy. You will be filled with calm and joy if you can just sit and take in natures beauty. It is a great form of meditation and healing, possibly the best because nature is healing in itself, oozing the love of life, wellbeing and serenity.

Be Alive, Look up and Live

Eat natural foods.
Now you have removed some of the nasty stuff that is put in front of you as food in your daily shop it is time to go back to basics. The purpose of this process is not to start a diet of any kind. The purpose is also not to deny yourself the foods you have been eating. The purpose is to replace the empty, dead and toxic food you have been eating with foods that your body will find value in, feel and have the benefit of, so you do not have cravings to eat, eat, eat as before.
If you are healthy now, great news, even so I recommend you consider what is set out here to maintain your health.
If you are having health issues of any magnitude, I recommend that you stick with the process set out here for as long as required to bring you back to health and then continue with it. This is so your

body can get over the addictions to sugar and wheat products (and I can assure you these addictions are very real) and start to re-balance before you start to add any of those things back in again if at all.

The more severe your health issues, the longer you stay on this the better. E.g., one of the followers of this process has taken the best part of the year to make any significant improvements in the health issues they had faced, state now that they will never go back to their eating of the past.

The purpose of this exercise is to give your body a chance to put things right, to re-balance and to start its own self-healing process. When it is okay to add other things, your body will tell you with its response. Listen closely and feel the response your body gives you and stop eating that which the body tells you not to even if/when your brain is craving more of it.

If you have a problem or reaction to any food remove it for a while so your body can re-balance. One way that you may get over small intolerance's is to keep off them for a while then introduce them in small amounts periodically i.e. once a month or so. This causes a spike of reaction in the body to the offender and over time will either cause a continued reaction or a better ability to deal with it. Sometimes it is possible to eat them again in small amounts later and sometimes not, so beware of what you eat and what your body tells you when you eat.

Remember - You must eat only the amounts and the types of food that your body response to best.

Where possible choose organic, although it is not as good as it should be because of American pressure, it is still far better than intensively farmed produce. And if you can get it from a local farmer and know it has had no chemical spraying, all the better

Every day, eat only high-quality food, and whole natural foods to provide an abundance of nutrients chosen from the following groups:

> If it doesn't look like nature made it
> and its not you that messed it up
> be very careful about eating it

Vegetables and some Fruit:

There is so much talk and information floating about on this subject that it is no wonder that everyone is saying different things and sounding very confused with what should be best for us to do.

For example, 1 to 3 a day 3 to 5 or 5 to 7 and 7+ to 10 a day. Just what does this all mean. Well it is supposed to mean the number of portions to eat each day. What is a portion, one potato or one pea, a bite of carrot or a piece of celery? Just what does it all mean to you because it confuses the hell out of me and every one I talk to about this it does them too when they get to wanting to clarify this point.

Let's forget all this 1 to 10 crap and eat mostly all vegetables in all of your meals with a little natural carbs and a small amount of protein added in, and when you eat as shown in the food Health Whispers Food Diamond below, it will reduce your risk of getting most of the modern day degenerative dis-ease's and improve your quality of life even into old age.

Also note that it is vegetables we must be eating mostly and only supplement this with a little fruit when in season and fresh.

To clarify all vegetables are a form of carbohydrate of sorts so when I refer to carbs here it is generally to the starchy type. It is also important to understand that with all things in nature everything it not equal, so different vegetables support different environmental growth in your belly and therefore support different areas around your body. Therefore, it is imperative to have a broad mix of vegetables to build a fully healthy being.

Now that is said let's get an idea of how.

Preferably fresh, preferably located grown, either raw, or lightly cooked, or in stews or soups.

Vegetables and some fruit should be more than 75% of your overall food intake. At Health Whispers we recommend you eat as many vegetables as you can every day.

Vegetables of all kinds can be eaten as much as you want and as often as you want, even to snack on. The more local, fresh and raw you eat the better it is for you. Any way you preferred them is okay so long as you eat them. I mean talking vegetables on their own and not mixed in some processed mess of sauces, salts and sugars etc. Remember you cannot overeat on vegetables and they will not make you fat, unless you do nothing else perhaps, so eat a varied range of them and not just one.

If it does not look like nature produced it and it is not you that messed it into something different, really consider carefully whether you should even eat it.

At his point I would also like to suggest adding in some fermented foods. Wherever you are in the world there seems to be some traditional foods that were fermented even if not so prevalent today. Like sauerkraut in Europe and kimchi in Korea. There are more good little guys, bacteria, in half a cup of them for your gut than most Probiotics you will find on any shelf. And if you make it yourself it will be fresh and live and satisfying.

More on the problems with the food supply in a later chapter

Carbohydrate: grains, legumes, pulses.

As stated earlier all vegetables are a form of carbohydrate so do not get hung up on that for that act and support you differently. What I am referring to here are the starchy carbs

Almost everyone I have worked with on this have discovered that they are intolerant to wheat itself and not just gluten. In fact, I will be bold and say that I believe that all the wheat grown in the west using intensive farming methods will create an intolerance in everyone that consumes it. If you do not think you have issues with gluten intolerance, then you are of the lucky few because you will have an extremely strong and healthy gut balance. But most usually agree in the end that they actually do have an intolerance to something in wheat even if it is not the gluten.

I recommend: - Rice, buckwheat, potatoes, sweet potato as better carbs as they generally come as nature made them.

Only eat the carbohydrates that are all natural and can be eaten unprocessed in any way other than something you do yourself like normal cooking.

This gives your body a chance to receive some possibility of actual food value to benefit from without the possible intolerance's and emptiness of wheat based and processed foods.

Rice I have found to be the best although this too can have had extra processing like bleaching: but it has other properties and benefits. You may find others suite you better so eat that instead.

Note: - One thought on rice and anything else for that matter, be cautious of anything grown in American as it is most probably Genetically modified or at least contaminated by genetically modified crops and is certainly intensively farmed and highly chemical grown.

You can also add in here things like mung beans, lintels, split peas, and other pulses.

If you do not think you have issues with gluten intolerance, then be aware of its possibility and observe your body messages. Although I do not believe it is just gluten that you are said to be intolerant to but other aspects within wheat itself like the lack of any necessary nutrients to allow our body to process it along with the intense high speed processing that kills what little of value that may have been in it. What's left creates a perfect environment or substance for fermentation of all the wrong fungi, bad bacteria, and rouge parasites to flourish.

Remember you are removing wheat to give your body a chance so do not break this step.

Also, more often only when you have stopped eating the wheat products and replace it with natural carbs for a while, will you notice how much better you are feeling.

Protein: Animal, Beans, Nuts, seeds etc.

Proteins of various types. Eggs, beans, nuts, seeds, fish, shellfish and other meats including broth from animal bones. Free range/pasture grown or wild and in its natural form wherever possible.

Note: These recommendations are from the consideration of food that we have naturally evolved with and avoid the processed and chemically laced foods promoted by the food industry. When it comes to food, know that natural is always better, and the more natural the food we eat the better our results we have for our health and well-being.

To get started all meals should consist of a range or combination of foods, i.e. Mainly vegetables with approximately equal amounts of, carb and proteins. Adjust the mix after a few days to find the portions of each that suites your body type best. See chapter on Fine Tuning and monitor your bodies reaction closely so you can increase and maintain your energy levels.

If you need to top up with a snack, then do so with the above supporters and not with a sugar or wheat-based product.

Nutritional Extras

Due to today's dead food and its chemical filled production, it is necessary to ad Nutritional extras/suppliments. Although the general projection from the big Pharma puppets, (the FDA of America) and the medical training of doctors is that nutritional supplements are a waste of time, this is not true.

If you take only the recommended daily dose (RDA or RDD) it may be true.

That is like running your car on E (empty) for only just about enough all the time and you know the stress this causes you when this does happen in your car let alone having that feeling all the time in your body. It is important that you take more until you feel the benefits of what you are taking. I recommend at least 5 times the RDA and even this may not be enough, provided the mineral content is either of nature or has been chelated.

Enzymes and Probiotics

These are both critical today if you live in the western world to help process and assimilate the food you eat and help with your gut health. They are not in the foods grown in intensive chemical farmed food nor do they survive in the high-speed processing, bleaching and heat-treated processed foods today so must be replaced. If you do not replace them your BAD bacteria can thrive by feasting on the dead food, you have no choice but to eat. They take over in your gut, causing even more health issues. This was something I did not realise when I first got fatigue though I did later have improvement when taking large doses of them. They are critical for today's foods and will remain so until we go back to natural grown foods.

Essential Fatty Acids. (EFA's) Omega 3. 6. & 9....

EFA's are missing from most people's diet in the west. Unless you eat lots of oily fish and avocado's most days you are not getting enough EFA's. This is the oil that keeps everything supple and working. It is more than just a lubricant it's also part of the building blocks and repair process. EFA's are an absolute must for health and you cannot get enough in your daily western diet. Imagine your car with no oil in the engine, it would seize solid fast. Well that's the same for your body but EFA's are even more important for your body to function properly.

Calcium Bio mix

The lack of the right mix of calcium is associated with over 150 different dis-ease issues and maybe even more. Don't be fooled by what you are told on TV, as you cannot get it from milk, and you must also take it with a mix of multi-Vitamin and Multi-Mineral to be able to absorb it for benefit. You know now that, that is not possible today as they are just not in the foods offered so until they are you will need to supplement your eating. The last research read by Health Whispers was Calcium Citrate and Calcium Malate were the best for uptake by your body, but you will need to do your own research and experimentation a little for the mix that suits you best. And remember they must be taken with a full range of vitamin's and minerals.

Glucosamine and Chondroitin

Are also missing and are most important for the joint health especially. As with Calcium, Supplement these and you will feel the difference.

Multi-Vitamin

Nature's own grown preferably, and this should include some Sun. Here we all have a problem, as little is left in the food we get so again, do your research to find what your own body responds to best by way of supplement's.

Multi-Mineral

Preferably minerals from nature's own grown plants or chelated supplements for better uptake. On a good day for you, Heavy minerals will give you at best a 1 or 2% uptake so most is wasted while chelated minerals may give you about 50% uptake and plant minerals about 90 to 95%. This shows the importance of going back to nature in the growing of our food.

We have a problem here, almost none of the food grown in the west today has anything other than some synthetic version of just 3 of the 70 plus minerals and trace elements needed for full and healthy function of both plant and you the eater of said plant, so again do your research to find what your own body responds to best by way of supplement's. Remember to get chelated minerals for better absorption if they are not plant based.

Flora balance - transplanting or transferring
One of the things we are all lacking today in the western world is a healthy balance of our little supporters and especially in your complete digestive and your waste removal system.
These little microbes are all important to your overall health. When you are severely compromised it may be necessary to get some from another healthy person to help you along.
Another factor in the west is our fixation on cleaning products, hand wipes and sterilisers to keep the bad bugs at bay however these things also tend to sterilise you of your good bugs too. It is better to have a good habit of washing of hands and use a white vinegar or a diluted mix of hydrogen peroxide which will kill far more bad stuff than those so-called cleaning chemicals you buy. They also strangely seem to support your good bugs, the ones you must have in abundance for good health. The point here is to wash your hands with soap and water and use these natural products to clean as you need and be less hung up on a few bugs about because when your personal system is properly supported a few bad bugs will also make you stronger. It is also very important to understand that bleach does not clean it just kills everything in its tracks including you and the environment over time. It does have it uses but use it sparingly and only when really necessary.
A thought to note here is that most third world people are much healthier with stronger immune systems than those in the west although we are told a very different story and yet we are consistently asked to support them by giving money. How will they support us when we realise, we are dying from dead foods and malnutrition just as we are so often told they are but for very different reasons, perhaps a faecal transplant from them to us will help us in times of need.

Food Rest periods
This is not based on any religious or fad diet ideas or any other crazy idea. It is based on how we have developed and evolved with nature throughout our existence.
What I am recommending is to reduce your food intake on your days off now and again where you can relax and not stress about your energy levels in that moment.

This is to empty out and rest your internal organs and body from time to time. It is always important to drink plenty of water even on these rest days.

If you do not do this your digestive system is working hard 7 days a week when you eat fully each day and never rested.

Have a day or two occasionally by reducing your intake to about 1/3 or less of your normal daily level to allow your stomach, intestines and bowl to clear out as many of the wastes and toxins of the week. I recommend you do this at least twice a month if possible. It is an easy thing to do, you could have a for example have a good vegetable breakfast with an egg or two and a little salad lunch, a small evening salad or you may just not have your normal evening meal. Better still make or get a green vegetable drink and have that on these days. You get the idea but the most important things to leave out on these rest days is meat protein and heaver foods because it takes longer to digest and therefor stays longer in the process and also Carbohydrates including sugars as these stimulate the fat storing actions in your body. The point is to empty out now and again to rest the entire body from continuous work. You need a rest from work, so it is wise to give your body and digestive system a rest too. In fact, research shows that a reduced, but quality diet gives you a longer healthier life.

It is a wonderful feeling when this happens, and you feel much more vibrant and again ready for a new start after allowing a clear out. When you do the rest days your energy levels will actually increase over time. My personal favourite way of doing this is when I can is to come home on a Friday and just have a small salad, a couple of eggs for breakfast Saturday followed by a small salad or green drink when hungry and maybe another later in the day again a couple of eggs for Sunday morning, then going through to a late afternoon Sunday lunch. The reason I like to do about 2 days is because most of us take between 12 and 24 hrs to pass what we ate so this gives time to clear and a little rest. If you take longer to empty out, then take longer. I have done this from time to time even for a week and have found for myself and those willing to follow, that your body works best when you eat well in the early part of the day and less when you are preparing for sleep so if you are going to forgo a meal then the last of the day is the best one to forgo as the body somehow seems to do a turnaround at night and concentrates its efforts to feed your brain when sleeping so it does not need hours of food work to do when it should be cleansing, repairing and feeding the brain and body. This helps use any excess that has been stored so it is a good fat burner too. Whereas you need to feed your body early for daily function and keep the energy going for hunting and gathering. Now if your focus is to lose weight or more correctly reduce measurements then reduce your natural carbohydrate intake to mornings only and if a reduced stomach is your goal then reduce you last meal to salad or vegetables and a little protein at least 4 hrs before bed ie earlier in the evening than you normally eat and have nothing but water after this and through the night till you have a good hearty morning Breakfast. Now you also know from this book that breakfast does not contain any serials or grains so it must be a proper breakfast with, you got it, more vegetables.

The rest period is still an observation in progress, but it does give some time to remove and rest the system as humans have developed to do over time.

Remember we are not "junk food man" we are "cave man" after all. Another point here again is not to get hung up on any aspect of these rest days, regularity and especially calories. Calories are a confusing and worthless measurement for food intake as shown later in this book.

Do a rest day or days when and as often as you can in your busy life. It could be weekly, biweekly, monthly but at least a few times a year with a full water and green fast at least once a year for several days even up to a week if you can. Remember each time you do these they are a longevity extender and is particularly good in the early repair cycle to help clear out the waste and toxins your body so desires to be rid of. And if you have an illness or dis-ease of some sort it may just help to cut that short and give your body the kick it needs to start the defence system again.

The more compromised you are though especially if you are storing excessive fat, the more careful you will need to be with this because you will have been getting little food value anyway so will already be undernourished without cutting out food. When I first went through this I learned that reducing one meal to a little green salad before I went to bed was best for me but you will need to experiment to find what will help you as we are all different. And remember to continue with your supplements as these are vital, you cannot thrive without them.

Regeneration - Review and tips

Don't be fooled by what you are told through the media on TV, radio, newspapers and online as most promotions are just the next fad to take your money and your mind off the truth.

"Nature's Own" Grown plants are those grown on fully natural mineralised soils and grown with no artificial chemicals, either sprayed on or put in the land or plant, nor do they have any GM modification.

Keeping to these Steps alone for 3 to 5 weeks or more and all the sugar and refined carb cravings will just fade away. Yes, you may well have been in the grips of the most powerful addiction and craving, without even realizing it but it is also the easiest and fastest addiction and craving to get over. You must be very aware though, that if you eat more than a cookie or a cake now and again your body may flick back into the addictive reaction and cravings to it again. This reaction against the food eaten causes a compulsive urge for more of it in your brain. It is something to do with how the chemical make-up of sugars affects the brain that makes you seek more even though the body is reacting in stress, trauma and intolerance against them.

 Keep off them and as stated above it only takes about 3 to 5 weeks to completely remove the cravings for sugar and today's dead wheat products too and start those feelings of great Health After Sugar and Health after Intolerance.

How good is that.

Also Remember if you are a meat eater you will most probably eat a lot of meat especially if you live in the west so this may be a good time for you to reduce the amount of meat you eat while increasing the vegetables. Proteins of all sorts are necessary for all our body functions as well as sustainable energy but generally we eat far more than we need to today. The vegetables are key to your overall good health, survival, maintenance and repair to get you and keep you feeling great. After all vegetables are most likely how our ancestors started in the evolutionary process as gathers before we learned to hunt so it stands to reason why they must be the base of everything we eat.

It is recommended that you stick to this process for more than 3 months to give your body a full cycle to clear out enough to even start to re-balance and repair.

In the case of our friends and followers, most continue having improvements after 2 years and more, so long as they stick with it and you will too. We all break away and eat refined carbs from time to time but we also notice their effects on us, especially if it's more than a spike of them now and again we get the reminders somewhere.

Notes from Grandma.
Grandma always use to say that when you are sick or out of kilter (her word for not feeling so good) then get a load of vegies, lentils and lumens along with some lamb, beef or chicken bones and cook up a big pot of broth and soup. Eat it over the next few days and by the time you are finished it you will be feeling great again. In the winter when its cold and dark and you are in the blues do the same or make a mixed vegie and meat or nut stew. It's so true and I still do this to this day and it sure helps raise the mood.
Remember tummy happy, you happy.
If you do not eat meat, then use good vegetable proteins for you must have protein for full muscle and brain function.
Grandma also believed in laughter not just for health but for everything in life and often used to say "laughter is the best medicine so laugh at it loudly and it all just goes away".
Whatever it is.

Congratulations, you have taken your first steps on your way to good health.

<table>
<tr><td>Whatever you do, do not stop now</td></tr>
</table>

On the next page is a better food guide.

It has only been necessary to bring you this because of the incredible idiocy of the original food pyramid which was designed for the food and pharmaceutical industries to make money from your ill health.
If you ask this, it would probably be denied but that is exactly what it has done over the last 50 years or so.

The Health Whispers
BETTER FOOD GUIDE

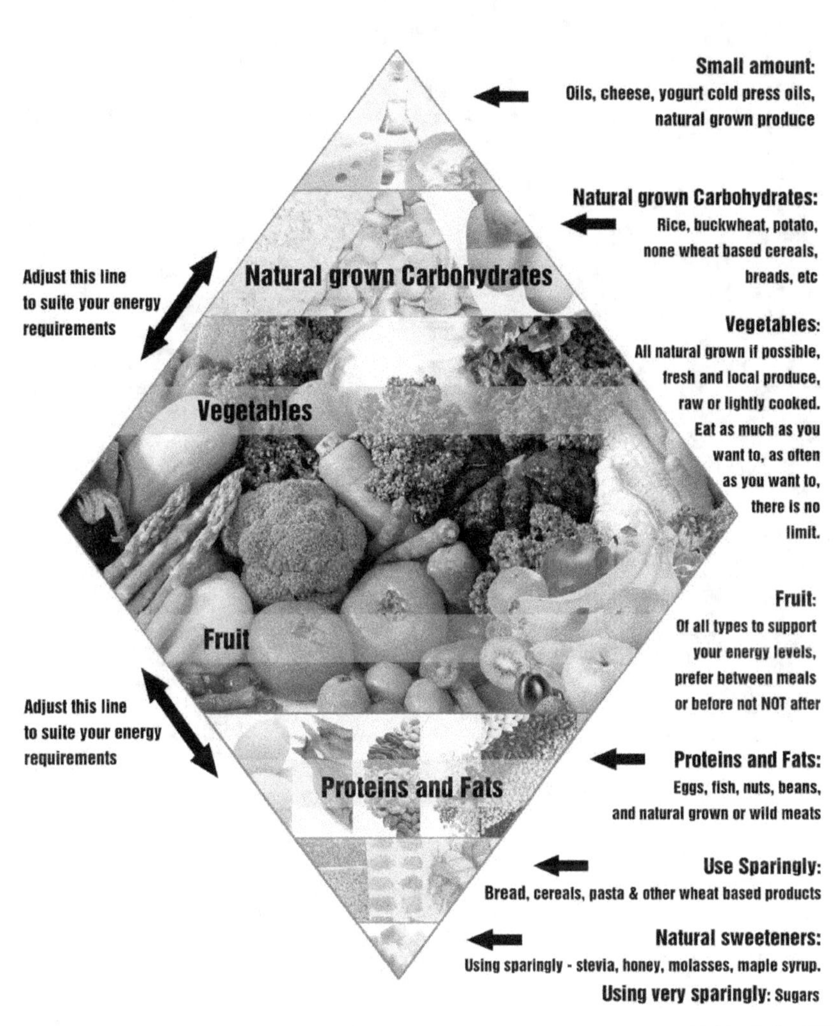

THE HEALTH WHISPERS FOOD DIAMOND

Do you really need all the excesses
To survive and thrive
Is normality and being average the problem
Holding you from
The fires of greatness burning within

6 ENTHRAL

Finding sanctuary, Fine Tuning your body bio

Before you get started on this, it is important to understand that one size doesn't fit all. Most things in nature are unique and this is especially true and even more difficult in today's mixed up and controlled world full of dead foods.
In other words, this section could be the most important part for your health, take careful note. The reason for the last two chapters is to heal your gut and get you feeling better and this one is taking it further to get the balance right. First of all your stomach must be acidic where as the rest of your body needs to be slightly alkaline for you to feel your best. Removing the offenders stops the damage cycle and taking on your supporters is to heal your gut. Together they are creating the balance and this section on fine tuning helps you keep it there right in your happy spot.
By feeling what your body is telling you and only putting in that which supports it. You will be amazed at how much better you feel and how quickly it can happen. When your stomach is happy you will be too as all physical feelgood health comes from the stomach. Only when you remove the offenders completely and feed on supporters can you be fully energized.
Yes there is all sorts of programs out there to stimulate your mind or to energize yourself and heal your body and yes some of them are good too, but until the offenders are gone your body must use energy to defend against them and to remove them or even worse when they cannot be removed they are parked somewhere in cells around your body and flooded with water to lessen their effect on you. Sacrificing those cells for the good of your body as a whole. The offenders are like rogue software coming into your computer, they try to screw it all up and your anti-virus software must work hard to remove or vault them. This is also possibly the reason why you are seeing so much cancer today because with so many toxins for you to contend with your body is so compromised that you cannot remove everything, so much of it gets parked inside and those cells to fester.

Although it is possible to clear and be unaffected by toxins by using your mind, this is not a reality for most. With the ever-increasing build-up of manufactured chemicals and toxins in the environment and food supplies today it is difficult to target them all so every day you are only a few steps away form a health crisis, so beware.

The following are guidelines only to approximate proportions. Adjust to suit your needs

1. Reduce or cut out all refined carbs and sugars altogether but certainly <u>less than</u> 5% of your total daily food intake even if you believe you are able to tolerate them, although I recommend you remove them completely for faster benefits and weight loss. If you have health issues removing them completely is essential.
2. Adjust your fresh vegetable and a little fruit intake to 75% or more and the natural/grown carbs to about 15% of your total food intake. The other 10% to be proteins of various types of eggs, beans, nuts, seeds, fish and other meats (preferably free range grown like grass feed or wild).
3. Adjust (as shown on the Whispers Diamond) the quantities of each to suite your own body's needs remembering to maintain a high level of a varied mix of fresh vegetables.
4. Do not get hung up too much on the quantities and never count calories but use this as a starting point or guide for the best approximate portions that give you the best results, especially energy. Adjust as needed.
5. To repeat, it is important to notice the reaction of your body on which food, mix or combination is best for you. Remember here that although your body is rejecting things like sugar the brain may crave it so only listen for your body response and resist the brain cravings.
6. It is also important to have some time out on a much-reduced intake to rest. It can be a day or two now and again or what you feel comfortable doing. There are no rules here, but you will feel the benefit when you do it.

On your reduced food day's the important thing is eat only on light and/or soft foods like soup or salad that support your good stomach bacteria and still allow your bowels to clear out the heavy stuff.

I find, and when I have worked with others, that about 1/3 of your normal day's intake works well, but again you will need to experiment a little to see how you feel and adjust accordingly. This is to give your body the time for you to clean out the waste and have some time to rest as explained earlier not as any fad diet concept.

For example, if you do not sleep for a week would you still be active and productive. The answer is certainly not, so why do you keep stuffing your body full of dead food making it work like crazy 24/7 with added overtime to clear up the mess you just stuffed down your neck to feed it and then wonder why you are not functioning.

Getting the balance right
There is much physiological diversity among people and therefore a broad spectrum of dietary needs. It may be that your body's requirements may be very different, from the people around you.

> There is no such thing as a general or generic plan,
> and this is certainly not a strict diet,
> there is no counting calories,
> weighing food or restricting amounts,
> they are all out.
> It is one you must customise and adjust
> constantly to best fit your bodies needs
> to both satisfy and stimulate
> while repairing it.

The personal mix that is best for your body may also change a little from day to day depending, as your biorhythms change but get your guide mix as close to right as you can and you will, with a little adjustment or tweak as needed keep your energy in balance.
I recommend to start a new note book to track and to reference your progress on how you are feeling each day and noting what you have eaten different when your body mood is down.
Do not rush the process but keep taking notes and reference them until your indicators, show the position that you feel best with, as shown below.

It is important to make notes before you start and each today and for a few weeks at least, of how you feel, especially in the morning before breakfast, just before lunch and just before dinner. If you do not have this reference point then what marker do you have to measure and see the improvement.

Getting this right can seriously help with all eating disorders and dysfunctional eating. It can also dramatically help to re balance the neuroscience aspects of such disorders. The hard part is, as with every new change you undertake, is getting started. Being hard headed and stubborn with yourself in doing this for the first few weeks is one way, but you will have to find your own motivator to keep you on track. Once you do get it going and you see that you are feeling much better it will be easier. So just get started any way you can with removing the offenders and agitators and eating your supporters. And it may be a good move to do this with everything in your life but one step at a time, right.

Print or copy the next page
From this chart you will work out where you need to adjust the foods you eat for your best feel good factor.

Your Chart

*Emotional

| 1 | 2 | 3 | 4 | 5 | 6 | 7 | 8 | 9 | 10 |

On edge   Best Calm

*Appetite

| 1 | 2 | 3 | 4 | 5 | 6 | 7 | 8 | 9 | 10 |

Less   More

*Energy

| 1 | 2 | 3 | 4 | 5 | 6 | 7 | 8 | 9 | 10 |

Less   More

*Carbohydrates   Protein

| 5 | 4 | 3 | 2 | 1 | 1 | 2 | 3 | 4 |

*Sugars/Wheat's

| 1 | 2 | 3 | 4 | 5 | 6 | 7 | 8 | 9 | 10 |

Less   More

Daily Water intake: in 500mil amounts

| 1 | 2 | 3 | 4 | 5 | 6 | 7 | 8 | 9 | 10 |

<u>Your balance indicator.</u>
Adjust the two centre markers as you find what balance works best

| | | |.

Carbohydrate   Mix of Vegetables   Protein

Note: - You generally only actually need a smaller amount of protein if it is meat. As nice as it is for the meat eaters the trend in the west is to eat much more than you actually need.

It is possible you have begun to eat more protein because all the other foods do not give you anything close to what you need to thrive, it is very possible.

The other option is to make your own charts showing your indication from 1 to 10 of the above in relation to Emotional calm, appetite, energy and whether your preference is for carbohydrates or protein and/or the intake of offender foods like sugars and wheat based foods and also those other foods you think you may have a reaction to however small that reaction may be. And most importantly the water you drink. Remember the most overlooked aspect to feeling great is water. As your body is mostly water it is vitally important to keep it topped up with this amazing substance. Aim for at least 2 litres a day and some of you may need more, even much more. Try it and you will see how much better you feel, it's amazing.

Keeping a chart is the easiest way to keep track of your body's reactions. Remember this is about what your body is saying not the story you think you want in your head. They are two very different factors as the story in your head is attracted and addicted to the bad stuff, the poison you feed it, while your body only wants what supports it to continue to survive, thrive and feel good.

Doing this each day when you eat then be aware of how you feel till the next time you eat again will give you the markers for improvement.

By doing this, and knowing what you ate previously will show you what your body's response is to what you are eating and therefore what is the best food for maintaining your energy levels and emotional calm throughout the day and through the night.

E.G. If you are very hungry and low in energy you may have been eating too much carbohydrate (especially if it's the refined type). Your body's needs may be for protein or real carbohydrate or more vegetables.

Don't restrict, adjust instead and your body will do the rest.

Initially you may need some trial and error here till you understand the message you are receiving as remember your mind and the trickster within and it can trick you onto believing that all this is a load of old tosh and all that old shit you eat is all right.

Then follow Your balance indicators.

Especially the mix of Carbohydrate, Mix of Vegetables, Protein.

Your body's preference point will be somewhere along these lines. The further to one side or the other would require you to eat more of the one and less of the other. Remember vegetables and a little fruit must be about 75% of everything you eat so the adjustment is between how much carbs and protein you need to keep the balance.

I.e. if you find your preference is to the left you may require more carbohydrate and less protein or vice versa.

Having said all that, there are a few people that function better when the carbohydrate and protein is not mixed. In such a case it is important to maintain the levels that you require of each, but you may need to eat them in separate meals or an hour or so apart at least. I recommend starting with the protein.

There is no mistaking that your body knows best what is needed. It will let you know very clearly that it needs more of this or that and will only settle or calm itself when you are feeding it correctly.

When you are not it will be on edge and sending out signals that you will most likely misunderstand as it is asking for more when it is most probably saying no more of that rubbish, I want real food. It is up to you to observe it well.

You most probably will not understand these messages you are receiving from your body in the beginning but you will once you actually start to feed it with the right food, so stick with it until you feel the benefit and understand the messages from your body.

With today's dead foods, it is extremely difficult to reach 10 on the emotional calm and energy scales but I recommend you always work toward such a feeling and the more the food you eat looks like nature produced it the better it will be.

No matter what your Doctor, Dietitian, or other health professional may tell you, your body knows better than all of them put together, what you need for its fulfilment and its up to you to take full responsibility to interpret them correctly.

Remember this is not a precise science. Your body changes all the time so by doing the charts above, you can get a closer understanding of the types of food and the proportions that work best. You will also get a better understanding of the foods causing intolerance's and cravings so you can remove these agitators.

What are you aiming for?

You will know when you get close because your appetite and energy will even out and be more constant. You are aiming for as high as you can get it, at least above 7 for emotional calm and energy levels however this may take some time. With your appetite being low throughout the day and only building as it gets closer to mealtimes. Without all those, must have craving feelings of the past may I add.

With time your carbohydrate, vegetable, protein mix indicator will become in a more stable balance as you adjust it to your needs. Note: For appetite do not confuse cravings for needing to eat real foods. There is a big difference. Real foods will last many hours and give a feeling of calm before hunger sets in as opposed to the dead food constant cravings for more.

It can be helpful to top up your hunger with some real foods like Vegetables and/or Proteins to keep you energized throughout the day. E.g. A bean Salad, a mixed salad, an egg, a handful of nuts, some dried fruit or some dried meat or any vegetable will work, like a carrot or stick or two of celery.

If you are still having problems however in achieving a good constant energy level whatever you do, don't get all stressed out over it, just keep adjusting till you get there.

If it's not working initially, go back to basics and start again but this time make sure you keep off the refined carbs and sugars. Like breakfast cereals, who's story is it that these mean breakfast? Not yours but most of you have bought into it.

You may also have issue with combinations of food.

As the body processes them as and when it receives them, one food may not be good with another. Individually they may be ok but together they may not.

E.g., never drink orange juice when eating protein.

There is another point to stress here. Your body works and functions in a truly miraculous, quantum way, far outside your normal human liner thinking, so the messages and responses you receive may not fit how your thought process function and can be in metaphor's, so practice will be needed to understand the messages you are sent. I have found it easier to work with the feelings and images I receive and that is why the charts are based that way. Eventually you will get the message if you keep practicing.

7 INVEST

In Your Understanding of Intolerance, Cravings and toxins, The simple truth to health

BE CAREFUL THINKINGTHAT ALL FOOD IS YOUR FRIEND, IT MAY NOT BE, ESPECIALLY WITH TODAYS MESSED UP FOOD.

Intolerance's cause sensitivity and cravings followed by inflammation and body damage followed by dis-ease.

A vital first step is accepting that you may have a problem with your health and therefore what you are eating.
If you don't at this time and you are feeling great that is really good for you now but remember that if you live in the western world especially, modern foods lack goodness for life, are generally full of chemicals from production and processing so can your good health last. I have found that it can be a slow build up within your body that you may not really take notice of or even realize it is happening until one day it may strike or slap you. You have a little, or even a large, health crisis that you wonder where it came from. This is just like filling a watering can, all is ok as it fills, then suddenly it cannot take any more, it overflows and goes all over the place. Your body reacts in the same way, resisting the toxic build-up in incredible ways in its desire to stay healthy until it cannot take anymore and bam your health is compromised. This is why you cannot be complacent in believing you are ok now and that it will always be that way. Don't be like most people and think "It won't happen to me" because it already is happening to you even if you do not realise it yet.
There are many examples of this
I recently heard of a Story of a man that suddenly fell ill, although its clear it developed over many years. He went to several doctors and got diagnosed from "We cannot find anything wrong with you" to "You have developed "calcification", "gout", "arthritis",

fibromyalgia (all are the diagnoses of different Doctors for his same complaint). This was showing with pain throughout his body but especially on his hands, elbows, feet and knees. He did say that there was pain generally throughout his body and muscles too, but the key thing to observe here is that this was mostly attacking the joints and the muscle around them.

Only one of the Doctors he saw asked about his Diet, in this case Die-t would be better. The die is self-explanatory and the t standing for today. What this man was eating, and drinking was all the things stated here in this book as the offenders and little else. All refined carbohydrate and masses of sugar fizzy drinks. All the things that kill the digestive process and cause acid build up in the body, putting toxins in that solidify, usually in the joints and are then hard to remove. The result or effect is that these toxins especially from sugar and wheat today always seem to end up coming out of the blood stream into the muscle and become logged in the joints, this causes a reaction and they settle for the long term as calcification build up. To keep doing these things is nothing more than self-torture so if this is anything like you, go back to Removing the Offenders chapter and stop it right NOW or pay the price of pain sooner or just a little later.

As I revise this to update things there is the best example of this Slow suicide. "Britain's fattest man dies at 65stone" at 33 years old. He ate 10,000 calories a day of dead food and nothing else and eventual the body couldn't take any more and in his case it all ended in death by toxins and malnutrition. Note the word calories and irrelevance of counting them in a die-t and the connection to dead food.

He was eating 10,000 calories a day and yet died from malnutrition and they say that malnutrition is a third world problem?

There was also a few years ago, the American who lived on refined carbohydrate. This man got to half a ton in weight and was so malnourished that when he had to be moved his organs were so fragile that any stress in the move could have kill him. A special crane had to be brought in and the entire wall removed from his house to allow his removal to avoid body movement. When they rolled him to one side just enough to get the platform under him his fat had formed a flat mass to the side that was laying right across the bed and stayed that way like a counter balance making it very difficult to move him.

The point is that these men had the greatest cases of intolerance to the food they were eating with their mind misinterpreting the messages of "don't give me any more of that shit" to "feed me more, feed me more", " I want more", "bring me more". The ultimate addiction.

The purpose of these stories is to help you understand the significance of where most people are today, due to the dead foods you are offered in your daily shop and the information you are told about food. Even if you yourself do not believe you have intolerance, I have found that most of us do. Even if the intolerance is small now, it may not always be that way. Be aware as they may rise up without warning like a giant serpent in attack.

Intolerance's and your compromised condition may appear to be small or insignificant or just the opposite. They may not show on the outside at all when in the early stages but as they grow, they get more severe, they may even appear as breakouts in the skin although this is less common today because the food is so dead. There may be as many reactions as there are intolerance's in people. If your compromise is in the stomach because of your dead food it may not initially show in your gut, there could be all sorts of other reactions from both physical and brain issues and pain in strange places anywhere around your body.

To do nothing about this is Slow Suicide
By Self Torcher.

It is important to remember however that whatever place you are in regarding your health, intolerance is trouble waiting to happen and extremely dangerous to you on the inside with your present-day compromised system, (body).

I hear your little voice stating, that you do not have any intolerance's. If this is true, then you are probably one of the lucky few. Most people in the present-day have some form of intolerance even if they believe it not to be true. This is almost guaranteed due to what you are told to eat and the poor quality of Food that is on offer to you in the western world today. Some other places are not much better either for chemicals banned in the west are still being dumped on the third world.

Remember

> Big Phama must keep the lies alive
> To keep making money
> by any means possible,
> compromising your health for even more returns
> making profit at your expense
> You PAY to play their silly game
> Of legalised criminality

It is also important to understand that there is no need in most cases for you to detox. Your body does this very efficiently when it is healthy but when it is dealing with intolerable food it may not be so efficient in this as it is so side-tracked in dealing with that shitty food that it does not want and feels is poisoning it. Better to remove the offending food or foods and/or drink and let the body take care of the detoxing. If you have been eating large amounts of wheat and dairy and your bowl is clogged and hard then a detox of the bowl may be of help.

What are intolerances?
Anything that stresses your body in any way internally.
Feeling a little on edge, agitated, Irritable, A feeling of nervousness, have bladder Irritation, have food cravings, especially between meals, but mostly just feeling uneasy Without being able to explain why.
This can be an odd feeling or slight pain in the stomach that is often confused as hunger, a slight feeling of irritation in any part of the body or all over it, like a warming, tingling, itching or a myriad of uneasy feelings anywhere in the body and especially the feeling that it is in or under the skin. You could have headaches or blurred eye site or swelling of the stomach or throughout the body, especially in the legs and the joint areas.
The more obvious signs are often, stomach bloating, skin irritations, swollen and stiff muscles and joints, to irritable bowel and much more.
Cravings are indicators of the bodies' memory of food, drink or other substances, seen or unseen that are harmful to it.

Well these are just some of the initial indicators of intolerance to one food or another or perhaps even a combination of foods.

Our note on why this is so important:

You have all been told by science and medicine that your brain is the holder of our memories.

At Health Whispers we believe that this is not true. It is just our theory from observations and there are not any indications at the present of real science or medical talking of such a thing as yet, but we believe they will be in the future.

OK so the way we see it, the brain is the controlling unit like the central processing unit (CPU) of the computer. The CPU on the computer does not hold any, let alone all of the memory, there is a separate hard drive to do that. In all animals (humans, being one of the animal species) we believe the same process applies. The brain is your CPU that receives and sends all of the signals for your body to function and that your memory of all things is stored in every cell throughout your body. You can see this in the wild where many animals know what to do at birth, it is in their DNA passed from mother to baby held in every cell. Withing minutes of birth their body is alive and ready to stand and run with the adults for survival.

 On the computer analogy your body is the hard drive or memory and the brain acts on the information it is receiving from the body and then sets in motion relevant responses to the info it has received. So all your body cells hold all the information and memories of the whole body and all its experiences.

Use the following analogy's as an example

If you apply this theory to Alzheimer's, is this possibly the reason why somebody with Alzheimer's can remember things from the distant past but absolutely nothing from the present. Their body, being the memory holder, is contaminated by dead food and chemical toxins and the cells that would hold these new memories are compromised so much and the receptors that allow access to these cells are also completely blocked by vegetable oils so nothing will pass into the cells. So, most of the present memories just float around and cannot be stored. Older memories previously stored before all this contamination of the cells and receptors became serious, may however still be accessible to some degree. On a side reminder it is interesting to note that dementia is now the number 1 killer in the west today and this has happened since the increased spraying of toxic chemicals from commercial aeroplanes flying over head.

Also consider what the people who have sadly lost a limb always say. Their memory tells them that it is still there and how hard it is to get around that. All your memories are stored throughout your body so even with the loss of a limb this information, the existence of the limb, is still being received by the brain from other cells. There is a another aspect and very good explanation for this concept. Our bodies are about 98% water.

If you have seen the experiment where the professor has water in a series of glasses with the last one having formaldehyde you may be able to visualize the idea.

In each glass he places a pig's heart. With some electrical stimulation the hearts in the water pump a little as in the body but the one in the formaldehyde is still.

Then the professor empties the water from the glasses and transfers the formaldehyde from glass to glass leaving each one empty with only the last one with the formaldehyde in it again. He did not wash out the other glasses but just refilled them with clean water after passing the formaldehyde through them. This left the residue from the poring of the formaldehyde from one glass to the other. The hearts that had pumped previously were placed back in the glasses with the water and the electrical stimulation applied. But this time they did not pump, they just lay still. It is considered that the water took on the residue of formaldehyde left in the glass and became like it in its entirety (in other words acting as if it was formaldehyde in the memory of it) thus killing the tissue of the hearts.

There are other experiments with water too, some with love and some with hate speech at a glass of water. Some of each was taken and placed on a coffee filter. When dry they were later looked at under a microscope, the water of love had beautiful shapes like a snowflake does while the hate water was gagged and misshaped. Search for yourself and see, it truly is amazing.

As our bodies are about 98% water so does it not stands to reason also the whatever poisons or bad chemical toxins you add to it that they will affect you in the same way as the Heart experiment explained above.

And even more significant is how you speak to yourself. This will create love or hate reaction in every cell as with the water speak experiment. Beautiful happy new cells or misshaped unhappy ones that fill with dis-ease.

> Love yourself for great health.

As with the chemicals, you are larger in proportion to the amount received each time you appear to handle it. You cannot handle any of it unless you do not receive any more toxins and are able to remove or clear the ones already there. In today's world this latter situation is definitely not possible so the toxins build up and up till eventually they fell you like a lumberjack on a tree (unexpectedly from behind most of you will would probably say) and then they kick you again and again while you are down.

> They do not catch you from behind
> or unexpectedly for that matter
> as you are the one that repeatedly eat,
> drink, put on your skin
> and continue to use
> all of these killing you slowly products.

Your bodies neurological makeup is electro chemical in nature and therefore is affected by everything you do, say, eat, drink or even put on our skin.

Deepak Chopra says

> Every cell is eves dropping on everything you think and say.

I believe it goes much further than this.
If you apply this principle, then not only are they listening to everything you think and say they are responding and manifesting those same things you said and thought.

> What you think and say are as toxic or beneficial
> as the food you eat,

hence, being right in the head is the first step.

Our Planet Earth

To take this concept a step even further, so too is the earth itself mostly covered in water, so to the atmosphere and is also electro-magnetic in function.

This is a big subject but we will one day find that our beautiful earth too holds the collective memory and the consciousness of all life here and so much more by way of interactive and spiritual energy, support and sustainability of life far beyond our present understanding of how things are, I believe so.

This surly brings Interesting and exciting possibilities provided we all live within the realm and love of nature, the true provider of all. Will it also help us have a true alliance with god, not the religious interpretation of god but in a spiritual cognitive understanding.

In the modern world you also have to consider other things outside of yourself for example electromagnetic waves put out by AC power, transformers, and radio waves of all frequencies. Such things as florescent and low voltage lighting, radio alarm clocks, TV, radio, mobile phones, wifi and many other communication equipment put out these waves which interfere with you own natural energy waves.

Consider the words   Electro chemical

Electro

Our bodies require about 1.5v to function at the optimum level. This is miraculously produced in conjunction with our very own planets magnetism. Because it is such a small voltage and of an earth nature it is easily dispersed, reduced or unbalanced. The sign wave technology of today is very harsh and destructive on the gentle nature of earth and your own electromagnetic field.

The other consideration regarding your electromagnetic nature is the idea that when a certain path is activated, or action taken, over and over again, some memory or form outcome is developed. For example, of cravings or addiction becomes etched into the recording like a scratch on a CD. The habit is formed, and the resulting response is predictable. To stop such a predictable result is easy, you have to commit to something else that is better. To help keep the habit from going though, you may have to set up a roadblock in the scratched electro path so the message cannot get through to be actioned. Or better still set up a diversion that creates a better response and results.

This really is the basis of this book. Think, commit and act better to and for yourself

In essence: -

Change what you think, say, intend, do, eat, so your body has better memories to work from so you can redirect your action for better and better results.

Chemical

Not the man made chemicals but those of nature. Your body requires a full range of minerals and trace elements plus all the vitamins, proteins etc. These should mostly be from a plant source as our ancient ancestors lived in connection with the earth and survived by foraging while our more recent ancestors thrived with a top up from the animal world. All the food of our ancestors was natural and un-interfered with, so the other aspect you need is to not have any added chemical influences on your bodies.

Example; Our ancestors did not have any of the man-made chemicals around that we do today. We may one day (in a thousand years or so) be able to better tolerate some of these other recent influences but for now they are extremely toxic to our systems and I am hoping that we get over the control by the few, needing for us to be poisoned this way for their profit.

Remember it is your body that holds the memories of what you eat and it is your body that send the signal's to the brain to tell you what to do. Unfortunately, you mostly misinterpret the message and supply more of the offender when you are being informed that you are in distress and you don't want any more of that thank you. The more you respond in the wrong way with the wrong foods, the more confused the message becomes. I'm talking here of your body mind interaction and not just your mind process of what you think you are thinking or think you should be thinking or even think you are or should be feeling. This is more of a feeling in your whole being of how you are, an inner connection.

Back to Intolerance

If you have food intolerance and it is unlikely that you do not at least a little, with the products and food of today, it is critical, to identify them correctly, and avoid eating the offending food or using the offending products on our skin as soon as you possibly can. Without technology, identifying foods that you are having a reaction to can take a lot of trial and error. We can assure you however that it is worth every moment and effort that it takes to achieve a knowledge and understanding of the foods that upset your system. You may go to your doctor but your doctor may not be willing or able to help you identify the foods that upset your system, because it is "out there" in medical terms and there is no drug they can prescribe to fix or disguise the problem. If there was such a drug, they would look more closely, money you see.

You may also be tested for allergies, but this may not show all the individual or combinations of foods that you are intolerant to. Whatever your doctor tells you remember your body knows best. Do not let that discourage you. Even if you are feeling a little "off" but cannot explain why, investigate it, for it is most likely you are suffering from an intolerance of some sort or another.

Do everything you can, to seek the identification of these offenders. Once identified, eliminate them from your bodily intake. This may be necessary for a short time or perhaps even indefinitely. Continuing to eat the foods that you have intolerance's to may cause many health issues.

The 1st health issue is an addictive reaction, which encourages you to eat more of them. This may seem strange but liken it to a mosquito bite that itches; you want to keep scratching it.

The more you eat the more the reaction. Just like the mosquito bite, the more you scratch the more it itches. The more it itches the more you scratch, and you become distracted with it and cannon think of anything else. You scratch and scratch until you damage the skin and surrounding tissue. Then infection can start. If this continues it can end up as a festering ulcerated sore.

The same applies to eating the foods that are irritating your gut because they affect your body in some way, but the effects are far greater. To keep eating them is like keeping scratching a bit, and may end in serious dis – ease, only this time on the inside.

7 INVEST

Eating these foods means your vital energy needed for other activities like the important role of the body to give energy, repair and rebuild itself and be in a place of prevention are diminished or even worse, may even be stopped.

The normal function of the body when the right food is available to it is quantum, meaning it happens naturally as nature intended while the effort the body needs to deal with problem foods is completely distracting to it. The energy to deal with intolerances is immense compared to what it needs for its normal healthy functions. The focus is completely on dealing with the irritation and all else is overlooked just like you do with the itch of your mosquito bites.

When this happens the important things like the removal of toxins and dangerous chemicals that cause the degenerative diseases like fatigue through to cancers may not be done correctly. On the other hand, the assimilation of the good food you eat may not be effective so you miss vital nutrients that the body requires to do its repairs and renewal of cells because your body is so distracted with scratching the itch of intolerance.

Whatever the starting issues
the end result will always be disastrous
if you do not remove the offenders.

If you do nothing else from this book, then make sure that you do identify and eliminate all the things of irritation to you.
This alone will transform how you feel and increase your energy levels dramatically.

START TODAY
You may ask "HOW?"
The best way I have found as with all the people we have helped is to go back to basics and follow the ideas set out in this book.
Carefully being aware of your bodies reaction when you remove or reintroduce any foods.
In this book we are mainly focused on food and its effect on you but there is much to consider when it comes to understanding offenders as they are all around you so look closely.
There is much talk in the media about the effects of chemicals on you and some even state that everything is chemical, even water.

All of this talk is just further misinformation to confuse the rest of you, so you don't really have any idea or understanding of what is right and what is not. Financial reward for the big food and drug companies is excessively good when you are all kept confused and sick.

Well it may be true that all things are chemical, but everyone knows which ones are beneficial and we call them supporters. You may have called them foods until now, but supporter is a better explanation. The others that most people are referring to as chemicals are in reality the offenders and for most of you it is much harder to really understand if they are alright for you to consume or not after all they are in your foods and skin care products now so they must be alright. No they toxic and/or harmful to you to some degree just the same? Remember big business doesn't care about you, that responsibility is with you

For example, a good intake of arsenic will kill quickly but very small amounts may be very addictive but not kill immediately as with cigarettes. The real answer is that if they are not as in nature's own grown then they are not wise to consume and may well be toxic. And yes nature has its nasty plants that can kill but we know this already.

All of these strange, contrived and manipulated additives are in almost every product that you buy today even in the natural food by way of spraying or GMO implanting. It is totally unnecessary for our real needs, but it seems to be desirable, for big business makes even more money on the back of your ill health. So much so that farmers and producers today cannot think of any other way to produce their foodstuffs without big chemicals and unnecessary substances. This is simply because of the information they have been education on.

The chemical producers have a lot at stake in this, for if the truth gets out and you spread the truths of this book so enough people stop using their products, they will lose their profits. This is why they keep their lies alive in any way they can.

We encourage you to remove as many of these additives and toxic substances from your life completely

Investing in your Understanding
Further Considerations

Add to these, your own considerations

Achieving your ideal food mix each time you eat will maximize your performance both physically and mentally and will also stabilize you emotionally. Don't concern yourself about all the calories and weight loss chatter or stress out about other health issues. Focus your mind on identifying and removing wrong foods, finding your ideal foods and achieving your best food mix and all the other issues will most probably start correcting themselves. This is not a quick fix process and does not happen overnight as it can take several months for real improvement. It is well worth the effort for when improvement does show itself to you it is real and lasting and not just a drug disguised misconception, its nature working for you. If you are not satisfied or feel some irritation after a meal or still have food cravings (especially for sweets) most likely your combinations are still incorrect or you may be eating something that you have an intolerance to, are reacting to or even allergic to.

Although the following is something for you to experiment with to gain the best balance for you it is important to keep adjusting till you get It rIght.

1. When you are stressed, you may need to adjust your mix and add protein.
2. Keep the charts going for as long as necessary to track your progress.
3. If your preference is toward protein, then eat sufficient protein and this includes fat (but not any of the heat-treated oils) at the same time as you eat your other food. This will slow down the speed of sugar entering your bloodstream. For Some people it may even be better to start a meal with the protein.
4. If your preference is towards carbohydrate, always eat your allowable natural protein at the same time especially if you have blood sugar issues.
5. The same applies if your preference is mixed. Eat whatever natural protein and fat is best for you at the same time you are eating your carbohydrates.

6. Don't get caught by the old habit of eating sugary treats after a real meal because it just breaks the cycle of benefit in your gut.

7. When you look at the glycaemic chart, you will note the foods that are low and those that are high. Low means slow release of glucose into your system while high means fast release of glucose into your system. This may be helpful in relation to the glucose released into your system but does not take into account or consider the other properties, benefits or harm that one food may give over another. Use this chart only as an indicator and eat those foods that are best for your body type wherever they come on chart with the exception of the columns, sugar, and dairy. You will find your body does much better when you remove these all together or minimize them to a very small part of you overall intake of food. Natural food like honey, chocolate, and wine have other properties of benefit so can be used in small amounts. Dairy is best to avoided all but a little butter, cheese, and plain cultured yogurt, and these preferably from sheep or goats only.

8. As long as you follow this process 95% of the time no problem, you could occasionally eat the things you used to, the treats like dessert or a portion of chips or finger snacks while out having a glass of wine with your friends. Do not waste your time feeling guilty just because you had a pie or piece of cake. Try to keep it as a treat, occasionally and that does not mean every day.

9. Only Look back at what is already eaten so you can look forward to what you can do now. Everything else is old news.

10. Do not skip meals. Unless this is part of your food rest days don't skip when food is needed. If you need a snack between meals, have a nutrition bar, a protein drink, some vegetables, bean salad or fruit or a carrot, some nuts, seeds or other protein. For protein drinks Hemp protein (made from the wonder plant banned by America) is best as it doesn't give the issues with intolerances. This is because it has no hexane, gluten, dairy, lactose or sweeteners.

11. Be very aware and alert for food intolerance's as they disrupt the balance and processes of your body and can bring on the cravings, addiction, lack of energy and even disease. When these cravings or addictions caused by the food

that irritates are not corrected it produces the need in your brain for more and more of the irritant food. Continuing with these foods that irritate are linked to excess water retention, reduced deep sleep, autoimmune damage and other issues, ranging from minor to extremely serious... Be very aware and quickly remove anything that irritates.

Because the foods of today are extremely nutrient deficient it may be advisable to add some helpers in the form of Probiotics (friendly bacteria), multi-vitamins, chelated or plant minerals, bio calcium, essential fatty acids (omega 3,6,9), glucosamine, chondroitin etc. You may need to experiment with this until you find a brand and mix that give you the best results. Keep trying as it is worth the effort. At the time of writing Health Whispers are exploring a range of supplements that will benefit that we hope to put out at some time.

Drink plenty of good water
The human body is said to be approximately 70% water by mass and some 90% water in the cells so it is not an exaggeration to state that water intake is most vital. It is possible for one to live for 30 days or so without food but survival without water and be able to come back from it fully is at best 5 days. Even 10% loss of water can be harmful or sometimes even fatal. And water acts as a natural cooling system, provides protective cushion for tissue, is essential for digestion and the removal of all the waste, it carries all the toxins out of the body, giving space for it to carry the nutrients and oxygen back in to replenish and nourish the cells. Start every day with two glasses before anything else.

Sunshine
At Health Whispers we have always advocated having your time in the sun. Apart from its feel-good factor of natural light and warmth, there are great health benefits from healthy bones to brain function and an amazing boost to your autoimmune system. The lack of sunlight on your bare skin means deficiency of what is known as vitamin D, however it is actually a hormone stimulant not a vitamin, and the lack of it is linked to a wide range of health problems. especially conditions like depression, degenerative dis-ease and low immune function and a 100 or so more.

Get a regular dose of sunlight or UV rays on bare skin. Beware to take it in small time chunks to start with until you get some skin acclimatization but even 15 minutes a day will give you great benefit and endeavour to get at least 40% of your skin bared to the sun whenever you can. If you have not exposed your skin to the sun before then only have a few minutes at a time to start with so your skin never gets burned and build from there.

Sunlight is very important to us as it is our main source of what is known as Vitamin D. It is important to note first that there is a much greater harm to you from lack of sunlight and vitamin D deficiency than there is from any issue you may face from sunlight itself. What you receive from the sun is one of the main ingredients of building a healthy and strong bodily system. You can only get the full benefit of this so called vitamin from the sun and the health benefits are many. It really is the sustainer of life.

If you cannot get out in the sunlight itself then at least spend as much time in natural light each day as you can. Artificial light does not give you all the required range of light frequency necessary for full health. Without it you may not get the full benefit of the food you eat either. You may suffer from procrastination and indecision from natural light deficiency or Seasonal affective disorder (SAD) or have such problems as headaches, fatigue, depression, anger, tooth decay, skin problems, ADHD, a range of degenerative disease such a compromised immune system and even cancers.

Note: To much all at once may cause problems also, not because it's bad, but because most of you have spent little time in it throughout the rest of the year so are not acclimatised to it, your skin is not used to receiving it and will burn and damage the skin. Your system is further compromised because of the dead foods you consume and therefore you do not get the other nutrients to build strong and healthy skin to protect you.

Also Note: Be aware, vitamin D supplements may help in winter darkness but do not give you all the benefits of being in the sun and to some people are said to be harmful and cause intolerance's in your body when synthetically produced. This however could be another ploy for you not to take them for you will be healthy.

Electromagnetic fields (EMF)

Wherever possible be aware of anything that may cause an electromagnetic field (EMF) as these disrupt your own energy field. It may be obvious that you should not live under the countrywide distribution pylons but you often do not consider the wonderful little radio alarm clock that sits on the bedside table right beside your head while you sleep. If it is plugged into the mains it has a transformer emitting EMF. This EMF disturbs your brain waves and stops you getting to sleep to a depth required to bring proper rest and repair.

You may also put your mobile phone on the bedside cabinet, right by your head at night, put it in the top pocket right over your heart or hold it for hours over our reproductive organs while you surf the internet. I have also seen women tuck it in their bra right against their breast and heart or under their belt of their pants right over your reproductive organs. None of these will end in a good result for your health. No matter what the industry or government say, mobile phones waves agitate your cells in unnatural ways that can only end in tragedy. Even government allowance is questionable as it is tested with separation while you all hold the thing against our head and often for much longer than any test. Keep them away from you as much as you can. Consider other EMF situations and do whatever you can to remove them from your living and/or workspace. Remember that the phone frequency is the same as microwave and you know what happens when you put things in one of those. The affects of EMF may be slower than a microwave in agitating food to cook but the affect is still the same in the longer term on you. With the 5G set up being installed now, it has the ability to enable the power to be boosted to 1k Watts and then there will be no difference to the effects on you to inside a microwave oven on full power. Why were these frequencies chosen when there are much better and less harmful ones available? For that you will need to ask the evil shadow controllers.

Oils

Use only cold pressed and mechanically prepared oils like olive oil. In addition, be careful when storing it. If possible, keep it sealed and in a cool dark place as light, air, and time will all speed the process of making it rancid. Also do not heat it as this too may alter the structure of the oil.

The same applies to nuts and seeds, as the oils in these will also go rancid with light, air, heat and time.
One diet does not fit all so eat the real foods in the environment you live to please your body.

Metabolising your food

Your body is genetically programmed to favour ancestral foods that were required to survive but more important to consider now, is the conditions of your own environment and the cultural influences as they have an immediate impact on you and your wellbeing.
We all process, metabolize, and utilize what we get from those foods differently.
It may seem a complex problem of understanding your dietary needs, but your body will tell you what is good or bad for you. If you follow the process set out in this book and then feel and note the changes, either good or bad, then follow the message you will win in the end.

Products "Healthy" or "Not"

Take no notice of those products in the supermarket that are marked as "Healthy", do your own research. The reality is that most of them are only healthy for the "Companies" profits when you buy them, but not for you or your own well-being when you use or consume them.

Calories:

Like so many things in this world all calories are not equal.
Do NOT stress yourself or get hung up on calories.

Calories are only a stress creator and a distractor
of the truth your body seeks
a worthless and confusing distraction
from what is really important.

When you eat the correct foods, your body knows when to stop, or when to ask for more. When you eat the dead foods of today your body screams out for something with value to it, but mostly you feed it the same old crap and it only finds sugars, toxicity and waste. Is it any wonder you are all so fat and confused when that is what you eat and your body is screaming for real food?

Meat
I have noticed that some meat from some locations affect some of us in different ways. Understand that it is probably not the meat in itself we are having a problem with but far more likely it is the methods of production and chemicals used. Be aware of this and monitor your own suppliers for more natural methods like grass fed. By the way meat is a wonderful form of protein for you and all the talk against it is just another aspect of the messages to keep you unhealthy especially in this time of all the other dead foods.

Low Fat is Crap
Stop eating low-fat and all refined carbohydrate foods as they will actually have you putting on many more inches or centimetres, pounds, kilos faster than you can imagine. This is because your body thinks it is getting food for benefit but when it finds nothing it comes calling back to you for more and more and more

Natures Own
It is important that all produce is grown traditionally without chemical additives, fertilizer's other chemical sprays and certainly not GMO'd which were initially and are usually produced in America but now forced on most of the world. GMO food is proven to destroy the immune system so avoid them completely.
We are told that gmo was produced to feed the world but this is a lie, it is to control the food supplies and if we agree to gmo food the world will fall into starvation quickly as they will never produce the seeds for you to grow nor could they even if they had that intention. Why you may ask have the same people built an amazing seed storage facility in Norway? to feed them when the food runs out. And you know what that would mean for you and me.

All local and fresh natural grown Vegetables and fruit, freshly gathered are what you need to thrive .

.
Some of the special foods to start with in no particular order.
Rice, Buckwheat, Unions of all sorts, Spinach, Garlic, Ginger, , turmeric and other herbs and spices

Apples including the seeds, All types of berries,
Beetroot, Celery, Broccoli, All Nuts and seeds, Chilies'
, Radish's, Sweet Potato's, Olives, Figs,
Banana's, Avocado's, Kiwi Fruit, Lemons, Cider vinegar,
Vegemite and marmite.
And many more too
Add your own to the list when you find them

Thoughts on Garlic.
Eat some fresh cloves daily with meals.
Garlic works wonders on bolstering up your immune system, to the point where it can fight off bacteria, viruses, fungus, parasitic invasions, and even tumour's. The medical establishment conveniently ignore, (as there is no money in keeping you healthy) is that your immune system when sturdy and healthy is capable of keeping the balance against and even eradicating disease of ANY sort. If it were not then how have we survived and thrived for millions of years. It was certainly not by hiding behind the chemicals from big pharma.

Dr Yoshio Kato, from the Oyama Garlic Laboratory, found that garlic stimulates the functioning of the mammary glands, prevents cancer, disinfects tuberculosis bacillus, lowers cholesterol in the blood, cures skin diseases, and eliminates parasites – among many other things. He found garlic to be SO POTENT that GARLIC JUICE, diluted with water 1/80,000 – 120,000 times as in homeopathy will kill cholera and typhoid and countless other germs. He also found that its antibacterial action surpasses penicillin by as much as 15 times.
Dr. Kato found garlic, raw or juiced, to be death to roundworms, threadworms, ringworm (not a parasite, but a fungus), and ankylostoma – basically known as hookworms. He further found it effective in cases of other fungus infections, pesticide poisoning, heart disease, pneumonia, frostbite, neuralgia, asthma, tonsillitis, paralysis, and even mental illness and will even help the removal of heavy metals.

Drs. Damrau and Ferguson, in a paper published in the Review of Gastroenterology, stated that E. coli, is prevented from making its poison that causes dysentery, when garlic is ingested with the meal.

Dr. Michael Jackson, from the University of California at Davis, researched garlic's effectiveness on antibiotic-resistant bacteria, and found that GARLIC has what he calls "keeping power". Bacteria and viruses DO NOT BUILD UP AN IMMUNITY to garlic. While Doctors routinely "up" the dosage of antibiotics, to attack bacteria and other pathogens considered today as virus, even though they do not kill these so called virus they just take out the bacteria they feed on, just to gain some degree of potency and effectiveness, In the 1950's, a dose of 100,000 units of penicillin was a very high dosage – NOW, several million units are common place.
Garlic is a miracle food. Used extensively for thousands of years, its healing powers are legendary. Even on the Great Pyramid at Cheops, in Giza, there was inscribed a record of the quantity of radishes, onions, and garlic consumed by the construction workers, for good reason.

Below is a list of some of the thing's garlic has been reported to fix or eradicate, through its antibacterial, antifungal, antibiotic, antiparasitic, anticancer, antioxidant properties.

- Cancer – Gangrene – Asthma – Allergies – Insomnia
– Beriberi – Arthritis – Cholera – Arthritis – Liver disease
– Blood clots – Heart disease – Ear infections – Lumbago
– Tuberculosis – Encephalitis – Skin ulcers – Pneumonia
– Meningitis – Worms and parasites – Intestinal infections
– Digestive disorders – Whooping cough – High blood pressure –
Impaired circulation – Multiple Sclerosis
– Parasitic diarrhoea – Excessive phlegm – Chronic colitis
– Lung congestion – Athlete's foot – Urinary tract infections
– Herpes – knocks it dead in the lab – E. coli – knocks it dead in
the lab – Infected wounds – Yeast infections – like Candida
– Arteriosclerosis – Atherosclerosis – Internal ulcers
– Inflammations – Rheumatism – Hypoglycaemia – Bronchitis
– Common cold – Intestinal gas – Strep throat – Emphysema
– Constipation – Impotence – Senility – Gout – Anaemia

– Dysentery – Sciatica – Gastritis – Diabetes – AIDS
– Typhus – Obesity – Angina – Edema – Fever – Hair loss

This list is by no means complete with what it can improve.

I have long since said at Health Whispers that there is nothing on this earth that does not have something at the other end of the scales to balance it out or neutralise its effects. That's why it is so important to protect the native forests and their people all around the world as they hold much of this knowledge and plant diversity.

Do we need modern medicine then, well yes it does have its place for example, when you break a leg, but not at the expense of the many other modalities and age-old methods that work within nature.

General Glycaemic index chart on the next page for your interest

Glycaemic index chart

General Glycaemic index chart

INDEX	GRAIN	SUGAR	DAIRY VEGETABLES	FRUIT
100+	101 parsnips beer	110 Maltose	103 dates alcohol	
90-100		100 Glucose 95 Glucose drinks		91 instant Rice 90 puffed Rice
80-90	88 potato baked 86 instant mash	95 sport drinks 83 jelly beans 85 pretzels		89 rice chex 88 white rice
	flakes	80 rice cakes	82 rice crispies	80 corn
70-80	78 fries 78 pumpkin 72 bagels	73 life savers 70 jam	75 watermelon 70+ snack bars 77 corn chips 72 Breads	75 Wheat cereals 75 crackers 71 millet
60-70	68 cornmeal pineapple 65 sucrose 66 beets 66 brown rice 61 ice cream 60 apricots 66 wheat muesli	71 pancakes/waffles 68 soft drinks 67 shredded wheat	68 cantaloupe 65 corn syrup 66 potato mash 66 raisins table sugar 66 cream of wheat	68 Rye –Krisps 67 67 couscous 61 honey 67 pasta/ spaghetti 65 rye bread
50-60	59 corn 56 sweet potato 50 buckwheat	51 chocolate 59 pastry's	55 mango 59 popcorn 50 bananas 53 yam	59 sweet corn 51 kiwi 53 oatmeal

Please note that this chart is added just to show you the speed of uptake in the body. It has no useful purpose as a dietary guide.

As you can see on the Glycaemic index chart, Sucrose has a low index and vegetable oils are not shown but they are both major toxins to the body while honey is above midway and dates and parsnips are at the top of the chart yet they are supporters and honey has other benefits too when taken in small amounts. Do focus on removing all the items except Honey, of Sugars, wheat and Dairy otherwise do not get hung up on this chart as it is not important to your real health and ends up as yet another stress to deal with.

Repeat - DO NOT GET HUNG UP ON THIS CHART.

Use and focus your energy
Not against others
But to create and manifest
That which fulfils you
With gratitude and grace

8 IMPACT

Shaping up, Put Activity into practice, Mind and Body

Be active every day in some way.

Exercise is another overlooked aspect to health.
The proportion of movement in your waking period must be comparable to the sedentary or seated period for good health and strong bones. Everything in your body is improved when you move your body, from bringing oxygen into the cells, clearing the toxins and emptying the bowl, strengthening your bones and the release of feel good chemicals into the brain. Even light exercise like walking, taking the stairs and standing while on the phone will help, so keep your body moving, it doesn't just burn fat, it helps the body to stay healthy and also maintain reserves of energy in a healthy way. It is important to understand that the more you sit the more you want to keep sitting but the reverse is also true so get up and move your body and stimulate the brain into wanting to keep moving to feel good.
Also building muscle is more important than you may think. Muscle will burn much more energy and therefore calories whereas fat is just a stored source of energy for muscle to use and with the modern diet all the toxins are also stored in the fat. With muscle you will become your own fat burning machine. Exercise that builds muscle is the key here.
There are many schools of thinking in relation to what you need to do regarding exercise. There is no doubt that exercise is important for, "What you do not use, you lose". It is important to exercise all parts of your body and your mind. What we have discovered, (And I must say are still learning) Is that short bursts of exercise 2, 3 or 4 times a week, mixed in with general daily movement can be sufficient to keep your body supple. The amount and type of exercise you do for your own best results must be discovered by your own experimentation. There is no need for equipment as you can get all the benefits of equipment from the weight of your own body when used correctly.

You might try, stretching in the morning, Wall slides or squats, Shadow boxing, Dips, Press-ups, Laydown Aerobics, Stair steps and stretches, balance and stretch, planking and more interspersed with running on the spot or Run lunges. There is so much you can do with what you already have at home.

For my own experience I find Non-pressure exercises like swimming, cycling, stretching and laydown aerobics to be better for my joints now. When I was young I did everything you could imagine an even loved to run, but following my health issues and the joint issues from sugar products (Even though I was a very light consumer) I find some exercising far too stressful on my joints. However, you do the exercise, because it is important to keep the muscles toned as this also helps the bones and therefore the joints. If you can walk or cycle about 3 miles every other day whatever your condition or pain level, you will keep moving for longer than those who don't. Remember it only takes a few weeks off your legs to loose enough muscle for you to struggle to walk. So much focus must be kept on keeping all muscles strong and especially your legs.

The same applies to the mind. Keep your mind engaged with a good book, a crossword or learning something new every day. Studies show that those who are watching Soaps on the television have less brain activity than when sleeping. You may be being Entertained but your mind does not have to do anything to achieve such entertainment. If you use the analogy of "use it or lose it", Is it any wonder that the Western world has such a problem with dementia.

Impact Tip - Do some body and mind exercise today
It will get the blood and oxygen flowing to energizing every part of your body

---

Its what you do that matters
No action, brings Risk but No results

---

9 IGNITE

Reasons, "WHY" & "What".
Tales from the edge, blindly being led
All is NOT as it seems.

The best advise you can take on board is to re-evaluate everything, everything you think is true, what you do, what you eat, everything. What you are being told and how you are being controlled is NOT as you have most likely interpreted it to be. Have you actually thought about how things really are?

Some Facts to Think about
What has been happening in recent times that were virtually unknown just 100 years ago. These facts have been taken in America and now the rest of the world follows close behind.

1. Obesity has increased by some 60% and more in the last 25 to 30 years.

2. Recent analysis has also shown that America has over 50% of its population significantly overweight or obese. This follows the sugar and low-fat cycles perfectly and the rest of the world is catching up fast

3. Heart disease now claims the lives of one out of every 2 Americans today, that is 50% of the population, two standing together and one dies, yet few doctors even knew what heart disease was before the 1920's. Incidentally almost all heart issues are not disease at all but clogged arteries stopping the heart from functioning and what is even more troublesome is that it is totally preventable. See notes on Vegetable oils.

4. Today one out of every 4 (and fast getting to 3) Americans die prematurely of cancer and yet 100 years ago this too was virtually unknown. The direct result of the effect of dead, chemical lased and sugar-based food.

5. Chronic and degenerative dis-eases significantly reduce the lifespan on average by 5 or more years at present and increasing rapidly. Degenerative means degrading and this too is from the lack of nutrition in the dead food. Today your body is not getting what it needs so it is failing in its ability to survive.

6. The status of cancer, heart disease, obesity, diabetes, fatigue related issues and many others, are now epidemic. Yet, just 60 or so years ago they were rare and in 1900's almost non-existent. This backs up the statement "Its genetics and not diet" as a myth and a lie and this make things even worse because doctors look at the wrong things to fix and miss the real issues.

7. Dis-ease of this degenerative nature is increasing rapidly especially among the young, including children with over 40% in poor health at the time of publishing.

Compromise the health of the parent
and the child is born, already compromised.

25 to 30% of **children** are significantly overweight or obese and this is rising rapidly today too and they may even die before their parents. Again, this was almost non-existent 60 to 100 years ago.

Your Poor health today is a direct result of serious dietary deficiencies, imbalances and chemical interference and all preventable if food was produced as nature intended.
As these changes have been introduced over the past 60 or so years, so have your health issues increased in line with it. This is clear to anyone following the evidence and now you know where to look to confirm this information.
These problems persist because we (here I mean WE, all of us) have allowed the Governments of the World lead by the American Government and its shadow controllers to lack the will to fix the problem at source because there is far more money focused influences and pressures to maintain us going down the road of

disguise, producing artificial chemical fertilizer, herbicides and pesticides and dead foods for profit filled pockets from ill health.

> Producing dead foods and the likes of GMO's
> brings extra benefits to the big corporate machine
> all from your ill health
> Money, Money, Money in their pockets.

As incredibly sad as this seems, it is exactly the way it is today

The addition of low-fat, diet foods and fad diets for example just compound the problems.
Then when your health issues start from the lack of any nutritional value in your food, you are only offered ways to disguise the symptoms with even more toxic chemicals, through your doctor.
And so the story goes on and on and on. You can fill in the rest of the story regarding this unhappy situation I'm sure with a little research and observation of your own. It is all so obvious when you look.
Perhaps you would be better to follow the info in this book and do even more research for yourself on how to correct these things and improve your life and those around you

Remember though to keep in mind: -

> They do not care about you and me
> Your ill health is Money, Money, Money to them.
> And control over you
> Now that you know, it's up to you

Wake Up, I beg of you, Wake up

When life is limited
When equality is missing
Living is much harder
Their normal
What is THIS "normal" anyway
Rather die free
than live in servitude
No more mockingbird
fear and scaremongering lies
Wake up, I beg of you, wake up

Learn how to learn
Think how society should be
Bring your ideas to the fore
No polluting or wasting the planet
Free energy for all
Now is the time
Stand tall in your power
All life matters
The safety and freedom
The future of all

10 EDUCATE

Some History, Fact or fiction
and Flying Promises.

> For a long time, a very long time
> the people of the world have been
> manipulated, brainwashed and controlled
> by and for the benefit of the few.

We have only to look at some of our known history,
Egyptian times under the pharaohs rule, the Persians, the
Mongolians and Greek and Roman periods, the Ottoman, the
various monarchies, the imperial Families of Russia, the dynasties
and communism in China, all of the elite monarchic European
civilizations, the Conquistador's and Colonialist's in more recent
history. All of the religions, especially Jewish, Catholic, and Muslim
religion's, right through until today's power brokers which I call the
shadow controllers and their Government puppets, you and your
family have been controlled, manipulated, divided and brainwashed
by and for the benefit of the few at the top, those in control.

Every one of them (except the shadow controllers for they had an
evil plan to conquer and control everything from the start) probably
started with zeal, doing the right things for a while, then they get
court up in their own delusions and addiction to power, "We are
God like" or more often "We are Gods", then as that spirals out of
control they deceive, manipulate, devalue and justify, default,
pillage, dominate and control. There has been no exception and
todays governments with their multi-national Corporations and fiat
based central money controllers are no different. They have been
in the default and pillage faze with a lot of dominate and control
mixed in and now the final dominate and control is under way. Just
look around you and you will see it if you observe quietly.
Be aware and be prepared, big change is just around the corner.

In today's world you exist but seem to be invisible.
This is because in the eyes of authority
you are no longer a sovereign individual,
you are just a number in their accounting system
A straw man to the corporate governance
so easily written out of the account, of life.

The manipulation over the past hundred years or so has been even more detrimental to your health, your well-being, your culture, and especially the environment than previously, even though prior to WW2 years they were extremely harsh times for most people.
In those early days, aside from the controllers and their destabilisation, life carried on in a fairly normal way. They ate the local food around them, what was available at the time and were manipulated by the landowners to do their wishes. The manipulation was harsh but very different than today.
The general conditions in which you live today, in the west especially, may have become easier but the manipulation is much more subtle and sinister.
The socialist agenda is the elites' story that you have bought into. It is unfortunately not as the slogan you chant of equality for all. It is full of heresy, hypocrisy, revenge, destabilisation, segregation, division on every level so they can grab control. And when they make their final move it may be too late for you and me.
Just look at the rest of the world since 1900 and you will see their record is clear, destabilise and war, remember you too can become missile targets just like they are doing to others. Agenda 2030, You slave you pay you die. A little research will find this to be true.

The 1st major adjustment that has affected you in an inner way (unseen and unnoticed by most but felt by the sensitive) was the changing of the calendar just a few hundred years ago from a 13-month calendar to 12 months. This may not seem like much of a change, but it takes our bodies away from the natural cycles of nature.
Where it really starts getting interesting is in the early part of the 1900's the shadow controllers made their first major move to take over the money system and set up the private central bank system. Who in their right mind could even for a moment think it right that

the people's money be owned and controlled by a private group, insane?

Then there was a group of scientists who researched and studied the process of our production of food.
This research was undertaken because in some areas the farmers were struggling to fulfil supply requirements, crops were not growing or were stunted and unhealthy.
The scientists discovered that it takes less than 10 years to fully deplete the soils of all its nutrients with continuous cropping of the same crop with no replacement of plant matter or cycling of different crops.
They went to the government of America (because this was happening in America) and explained the necessity for replenishing and feeding the soils with all the minerals required to ensure healthy plant growth, which was to feed to soils with the full range of minerals, about 70 main minerals and many trace elements too, some 90 ish in total.
The government of the time, (this is the 1920/30's), decided that to replenish the soils fully would cost too much money, remember who was advising them, so under pressure from the developing chemical companies that another method should be found. They instructed another group of scientists to find the least possible number of nutrients that could be applied to make the plants look lush and healthy and supposedly cost significantly less than what the previous scientists were proposing.

Does changing, avoiding or erasing
the question or the history
Bring you the right answer, Or fix the problem
NO
It takes facing up to the questions, the history.

You may (or may not) know what the new scientists came up with. They decided that out of the 90 or so needed only three minerals would be enough to have the plants "look" good and the term intensive farming began and only used these three, NPK for crop production since that time. This fertilizer has been produced in the synthetic or chemical form and can only feed the plants, not the soils. Note the benefit to the chemical companies here as they took on the job to produce these synthetically. With this method the actual depletion rate of soil goodness increased further with the use of chemical application/contamination, this is known as intensive farming today but should be called "doom" farming because eventually food will just not grow. With completely dead soil, is it any wonder that the food grown on it is also dead.

This is made clear by the following:
Apply too little and the plants are stunted. Apply too much and the plants are burned by the chemical overload. The 3 nutrients are nitrogen, phosphate and potassium. This makes plants look lush and healthy, but I can assure you that they are not. In both cases insect and fungal overgrowth explode to remove and break down the unhealthy plants for recycle, and that is all of the plants grown this way.

Incidentally the very same is happening inside your digestive system and your body when you eat these dead foods. The good for you die from lack and the bad for you thrive on the dead food.

The 1st group of scientists were horrified and stated "If we do not feed the soils properly to enable healthy plant growth as proposed (and not just feed the plants as the others were proposing and therefore as we do today) then we predict that within 50 years there would be a major outbreak of degenerative type disease in the population".

What is the real truth of degenerative disease today – Yes, the outbreak long since happened and now there's a major problem with health of epidemic proportions of degenerative nature. It's not a disease that is attacking you from outside but a dis-ease from the lack on the inside of anything to even sustain or maintain you let alone thrive. Stress too is another sign of this and doctors today do not recognise the physical issues in front of their eyes.

Just the lack of proper calcium alone (just one of the 70+) is related to at least hundred and fifty different issues that you face and suffer today. (Side Note; You cannot get it from cows' milk even though you are told constantly you can)

Vitamin E improves your chances of not having a stroke by somewhere near 70% whereas what the doctor gives you from the chemical Co has between half and 1% possible benefit with a long list of direct effects which they somehow call side effects. (Side note; stop the veg oil and this will avoid any possibility of blocked arteries, add Vitamin E and strengthen all tissue.)

Vitamin D, which you mostly get from the sun, is absolutely essential for body health and of course how you feel, your mood. Yet you have been told for years to keep out of it. Why? Because if you are healthy you may begin to think for yourself and stop buying their crap and no longer believe their lies.

Vitamin C, like all other vitamins and minerals you are told to only take the recommended daily dose or amount. This is to keep you running on empty where as some 5 to 10 times the RDA would be more appropriate and Vitamin C has been proven to be safe up to the point of bowl irritation which could be 40,000mg orally or 100,000mg intravenously. The results of which have miraculous affects against most disease and restored health within days.

What do you see today; almost all of the health issues of today are degenerative. From heart disease, cancers, strokes, sugar diabetes to all of the other joint issues, fatigue, muscle pain, Fibromyalgia, Parkinson's, ME, MS, and motor neuron and many more labels the doc can put on you.
I could go on, but it is clear from just these few, that the story you are being told in the official line is certainly, sadly, and most definitely not for your benefit.
The information here is to educate you about how food is produced today. And why only three mineral nutrients are used can be found in the library of Congress, Washington DC in the USA.

At the time of this happening America had shouldered, pushed and projected its way into being considered one of the top nations of the world so whatever America did the world tends to follow or more correctly to support their international corporate organisations, forced upon the world . Unfortunately, those in the American government today expect they can do this with even more forcefulness.

Don't get me wrong, I love America and have many friends there too but the shadow controllers have definitely got in control and everything else is now out of control while you pay in every way.

This is a big story to much for this book and all about manipulation of the narrative to divide you and me for political power.

The incredible thing about this idea of how to grow our food is that the process of using 3 nutrients in the production of food was very quickly found not to work very well. Because the plants looked great, they persisted but they were in reality very unhealthy.

It quickly became clear that there was a necessity to develop even more chemicals to help the unhealthy plants along. Because the plants were so unhealthy, spraying was deemed necessary to kill the fungus and insects that were attacking them. With so many unhealthy plants around to be recycled by nature, fungus spread and the insect populations exploded.

If you know anything about the eco system, you will know that fungus and insects have evolved as an environmental balance to breakdown and remove the unhealthy and dying vegetation. Just like the wolf and the lion take out the weak of the animal world.

Even then the insects and fungus do the final clean up

Is it any wonder we have had an over explosion of fungal, bacterial and insects in our crops where they are grown with only three synthetic nutrients when the plant needs the 70+ of nature?

This was an amazing windfall for what are call the chemical companies of today because not only were they producing the fertilizer, now, they were tasked to produce the chemicals to kill the bugs and the fungus attacking the plants that were unhealthy because of the lack of any real mineral value in the fertiliser which they also produced. A huge win, win situation that grew them into the big pharma, the out of control monster they are today.

What a money-spinner it all turned out to be on the back of lies so why not keep it going?

There is another and even more disastrous consequence of using these cocktails of chemicals on the land and that is the killing of the natural bacteria in the soil. Without these little friends there is no natural cycle of breaking down and recycling for plant survival let alone for plants to thrive.

Think again here of your gut and digestive system
for it is a mini farm just like the land, when you put the food
produced with these chemicals in it and drink the water filled with
bleach or sugar it too will lose the natural bacterial balanced
and grow fungi, bad bacteria and even parasites and you will
become very unhealthy.

It does not stop there though.
With this introduction of chemicals, the farmers of America started
to collapse and drop (like flies caught in fly trap) with a very strange
issue that just struck them down, supposedly out of the blue with
varying severity from fatigue to full paralysis. No one seems to put
the connection together but those supplying the chemicals knew
full well what was happening. The fly spray analogy and dropping
like flies is so apt. This new so-called disease they called **Polio**.
Could this chemical overload of this new problem which today is
even more toxic, be the cause of many of your health issues today.
Yes, is the simple answer.

You may not know that polio is an American disease, called so
because it started there although they love to tell you its been
around for millions of years. Not caused by a virus as you have
also been told all these years, (see notes on virus) but by toxic
shock caused by the initial introduction of agricultural chemical
fertilizers, herbicides and pesticides. Whole communities were
affected where these chemicals were introduced, there were no
precautions in place or safety equipment in those days, and no
previous exposure or resistance to such things so the reaction was
extreme. This same reaction also spread around the world's people
as these chemicals were introduced to other places, countries and
cultures, supposedly in the name of progress. Progress for who
you may well ask? Certainly not for humanity.
Over time, the shock has become less obvious in the short term,
but the end results are still the same when you look at the health
issues showing up today.
Unfortunately and allegedly the president of the day had been lied
to about the cause and told it was a virus and had backed the
vaccination because of the severity of what was happening to the
farmers and their families and he too was said to be affected.

Because of this, the lie was maintained and from that lie the whole world was vaccinated with the polio vaccination. The initial vaccines were produced on live monkeys and with this, another catastrophe for the human race, because it means that a whole generation, all of the people vaccinated in the early period of this lie now have a great potential to contain monkey diseases of great toxicity to the human system by bringing them into you directly from monkeys in the vaccine. Could this also be the direct introduction of other great sufferings to the human race?

The Polio vaccine like so many of them, is contaminated with cancer causing substances was administered to 98 plus million Americans between 1955 and 1963 and hundreds of millions more around the world. It's hard to beat this one for crimes against humanity in the contamination of the people of the world on any level, a silent killer inside of you, administered by the so trusted medical professional for the benefit of big Pharma. The US government and Dr albert Sabin were aware of the dangers of the vaccine since 1960 but didn't warn the public or call back the vaccine, and do not even to this day. Instead they let that batch be used up on the populous, most of them children and then produced more to contaminate the populous of the rest of the world, you and me. This program of toxification through vaccination is even more sinister today and its now being forced upon you by laws, statutes and misinformation for pair pressure and ridicule by the uninformed. Don't you be one of the uninformed, believing their lies and misinformation.

Not a good result for humanity and it also brings into question how the vaccinations of today are produced and what are they for? At Health Whispers we do not believe they are produced for the peoples benefit so just what are they for? One thought put forward to us is that it is keeping the myth alive that they have benefit (but that benefit is only to big pharma and the controlling elite, not you) and for the purpose of controlling the populous in times of unrest. Can this be true? Unfortunately, and sadly it seems possible when you really take a close look at things today. Note here, the forced vaccine program has heated up in America, UK and other countries in the last 10 years or so, are they expecting unrest and if so, what have they planned to do that will bring such unrest. This could be in the making but the reality is that most vaccines do not fix any issue they are alleged to fix and just add more contaminants and toxins to your already overloaded and compromised body and weaken your immune system even further. And Vaccine's soon will also contain sterilisation and a microchip for their total control.

And now Incidentally the World Health Organization (WHO) can quite safely state that polio has now been almost eradicated throughout the whole world. Great news, right? Not really because Polio is now just called other things like Fatigue, Fibromyalgia, ME, MS, Parkinson's, motor neuron and many others. All neurological issues caused by chemical toxic overload. Also where there are new breakouts of it you will find that it is in areas recently plied with new chemicals of one form or another that previously had had little contact with such contaminates or the doctors call it so because they do not have all the new information on the up graded naming's for it.

Perhaps it's time to add that it has been stated that this disease only attacks humans. That was easy to say in the early years, as there were no considerations given in any way to the animals and insects. The fact is the insects and animals were desired to be killed by such chemicals. Therefore, this was never considered relevant. Today we have another manipulated story told to us, and it is that the pesticides are specific. In other words, they only kill certain insects or Fungus or Bacteria that are targeted to be killed. That herbicides become inert when they hit the ground and only kill the plants sprayed or even only those intended.

What nonsense will you be asked to believe next?
If only it were that precise and/or so simple.
With big phama everything is sleight of hand conjuring tricks.
Consider what is happening to the Bee populations around the intensive farmed world.
The story is they are dying by 60% each year due to farming methods and especially the loss of wild flower habitat.
Their loss of habitat is bad enough but this sad truth is only happening in those areas that are using excessive amounts of agricultural chemicals from fertilizer to herbicides and pesticides and one might add the situation has worsened with new chemicals

i.e. intensively farmed areas are sprayed excessively in the hope of controlling the balance in such an unhealthy Eco system.

Imagine that for a moment,
humans controlling nature
By using toxic chemicals.

In the area's that do not intensive farm with such chemicals, the bee populations are reasonably stable and develop normally. Even in cities with much vegetation and parks (like London, NY and Paris) the bee populations are reported stable whereas just outside these areas where intensive farming takes place they are not. This is because of the types of chemicals being used on the farms not used elsewhere on top of the extensive wild flower and habitat loss. They may not have a scientific answer to satisfy the official line but is it not just so obvious? I ask you to consider whether this die off of the Bees could be **Bee Polio** (chemical toxic effect) that is causing the bees to just fly off and never return to the hive because they lose their orientation, or maybe even be able to return only to die at home or nearby from all out fatigue. This fatigue is from the neurological effects that the chemicals are having on the bees just like the effect they had on the farmers when first introduced and now on you today. The official line is not to say anything against the chemical companies (as they have so much power and money to lobby governments) and they themselves of course state that it's not caused by them, so we, the great gullible, must just believe what the self-appointed expert says.

We do not agree with their story or that they are experts, after all we now know them as expendable dependable's of the controllers.
Watch this story carefully.
Remember they have lied about everything else
why do you think this time would be different?
Why do you imagine that you are not affected by these practices?
Like the Bees, the impact on you is showing to be just as severe
As thousand die silently and painfully every day around the world.
You eat at the end of the food chain so you get it all.
What they do today, out there, hits you tomorrow or the next day
Are you blind, deaf, gullible or easily lead?
Perhaps all of them.

10 EDUCATE

If you do not wake up and join together on mass for better methods, humanity is subject to a sorry decline and early Death

You eat at the end of the food chain so you get it all.
Share this information quietly with as many as you can
Saving the bee's also saves humanity
Stand together and speak up
Till we can shout it from the hill tops.

This is not limited to the bee's, there are many other signs and studies that show the problems of chemical use or more correctly misuse.

One such study is on the alligator's in the Florida everglades. Their numbers dropped quickly over a few years and are now close to being considered endangered. They are still breeding but only at about 20% the normal rate. The real problem is that only about 10% of those being born are male and these males also have greatly reduced fertility. This is believed to be caused from the chemical runoff from all the farming upstream pouring into the glades into concentrated amounts. The glades are a concentrated example of what is happening to the land, to the animal population and therefore to you.

Don't just take my word for it do your own research as there are many other studies which clearly show the effects of modern-day chemicals on wildlife and humans.

You may say what has the everglade wildlife got to do with human health, well it has everything to do with it as the chemical runoff into the everglades is the chemical concentrate of what you are receiving in the foods you eat daily.

For example, you can parallel this with our own human story and knowledge that the human sperm rate is some 50% to 75% down on 1950's levels and woman are struggling more and more to conceive, all in the same time period of increased use of artificial chemical contamination of the world. It's not a coincidence.

I ask you to think about, what has changed throughout the last century to cause such a drop in fertility and such massive increases in degenerative dis-ease?
It is the introduction of what we call chemical farming or farming with chemicals and the everglades are a concentrated or speed up example of what is happening to the rest of us daily.
It is the example of the canary in the coal mine
and it is clear that it is dyeing,
we have to get out of these practices fast.

These are just some of the stories kept quiet under the official line and you know now the reason is to protect Big Phama, Business, their profits and power.
It is important to Remember however, that Natural chemicals are sometimes good, but they are seldom brought to our attention unless there is a company or organization that can see a financial gain in promoting them. As nature itself cannot be patented, legalised or controlled by any one company, (although there are many cases of American companies trying to do this) so there is no reason to promote it.
This is the very reason why there is so much manipulation of the environment and production of artificial everything in the place of nature is because it can be controlled and monetised.
This is also the reason for all the frensy to set up free trade agreements and pacts around the world. Free for big international corporations but you as the little country have to pay with your people's blood in return for allowing big corporate in.

To go back to vaccinations for a moment It can also be observed without much effort that the vaccination program did not stop with polio.
You are told and most of you believe
(with your hands over your eyes and your thumbs in your ears) that vaccinations are a means to preventing disease.

Is this true or is it just another myth you have been fed for the financial continuum of the chemical companies and the purpose of control by unethical governments.
Following the wonder of people blindly excepting being vaccinated against an alleged virus that does not exist, is it not possible that

the pharmaceutical companies and chemical companies could
have just created other vaccines in the pretence of controlling other
diseases, or even making up diseases for the purpose of profit. Is
this just another windfall for the chemical companies that you, as a
taxpayer must foot the bill for, with not just your wealth but also
your health.
The most truthful observation is that there is a lot of evidence, in
fact mountains of it, of the toxic effect of these vaccinations on the
body but there is no real evidence that this myth actually controls
disease. Because it does not.

> You are not being infected
> you are being affected
> what reason is there to vaccinate the healthy
> when treatment for the sick is all that is needed.
> Vaccine's are more toxic than worry
> Worthless effort against a non-existent happening
> Filled with cancer, A crime against humanity
> while
> prevention and Treatment are the real path
> Action to repair those actually affected
> Truth in support of humanity

There is however a lot of evidence that good clean water,
sanitation and personal hygiene is what really is preventing disease
and disease outbreaks. One only has to look across the world to
the various different cultures, standards of living and availability of
these services to see that this is true.

There are also some very interesting observations to be
made in the western countries with good water and sanitation.
When personal hygiene, especially proper washing of hands after
toilet use, is lacking as it is in France and the UK, the outbreaks of
infectious diseases like hepatitis are significantly higher than in
those locations that have higher personal hygiene standards.
So always keep up your personal hygiene habits. It not only
protects you it also protects others.

Now let's look further

Is high blood pressure and cholesterol really the cause of heart attacks and strokes or is it just the effect or indicator of another very real cause. See the notes on vegetable oils, sugar and wheat products. Could the combination of these so-called foods really be the cause of heart attacks and strokes while the high blood pressure and of course high cholesterol are only indicators of the possible results (heart attack or stroke) of eating such bad foods. Note the word Heart "attack", it is no such thing it is the spasm affects of blocked arteries and the heart goes into violent spasms without the blood flow because it needs blood to pull and push around your body for its own function and desire to stay alive.

It is so strange that modern medicine only looks at the last thing on the list as the something to fix and never seems to be able to go back down the chain of events to find the real cause.
Silly me, I momentarily forgot that modern foods and the medical profession is not designed to keep people healthy and not to keep making money for all those involved by keeping you ill and your desiring for quick fix pills are profits at any cost.

It is interesting to note that in the early part of last century there came a product, considered wonderful, introduced to the world called Coca-Cola and of course, all the other sugar filled soda drinks, that have followed.
If one overlays and follows the graph from the introduction and the increase in consumption of soda filled sugar drinks with the graph of the increase in adult onset diabetes and you will see there is a direct correlation and they run up in parallel, like 2 tracks of a railway line in an upward direction. It should be called sugarbetes. Note this also applies to the obesity graph and there is a further increase of both diabetes and obesity following the low-fat scam which are other factors to be considered too.

Then there was a waste product in plentiful supply and the big industry need to dispose of it. It was found to make thing taste sweet so why not put it in the soda drinks and dispose of it through the people. What a great idea and this is of course the deadly aspartame. Aspartame may even be more toxic to the human body than sugar, based on the research you can find readily.

Now we have all been told for years to only use vegetable oils of some form or another. That they will help avoid us getting fat and therefore also avoid heart disease. At less than a buck a bottle to produce it is a great product to promote and make money from. In reality these products are very different and harmful when ingested. Just think about it for a moment.

The oil from the seeds or vegetable plants in its original state has to be good for you, but in the present production of them they are not, because they are processed, heat treated and enhanced so much that after this they have to take the awful rancid smell out of them so you will even consider using them.

This processing and heat treating destroys the natural state of the oil completely and turns it into something resembling liquid plastic. All that is needed is the setting agent to change its state and make it more like a container or carrier bag. When you ingest it then you set that process into action with the oxygen in your blood and it hardens into a sticky gluey mess inside your arteries and anywhere else it can settle.

That is exactly what happens inside your veins and arteries. It becomes sticky and hardens around them. First blocking your processing receptors so you cannot properly absorb, release or filter the residues of food you eat (e.g. sugars and cholesterol stays in your blood with nowhere to go) the pressure builds in the blood and then the heart issues follow when the blockage fills your arteries.

When some of this hardened plastic like crust breaks away from where it stuck inside your arteries, it floats merrily toward the veins until it gets to the small tubes of the brain and Bam, stroke time. Are you a plastic man or bag lady?

NO, you are NOT, but the choice is yours to be or not to be and how you want to spend your last days before you go.

Living through a heart attack or stroke is harrowing enough as the supporter but actually having one and having to go through that is one of the most harrowing experiences of all. This I know to be true as I have supported several of each and the few that have come out the other side enough to explain the experience, their story is horrific adding to the inability to do anything but just about exist.

To clarify, polyunsaturated and trans fats, found in vegetable oils, margarines and any products containing these artificially changed fats are out and should not be used or ingested at all, NEVER.
Use the vegetable oils only for oiling the door hinges of your house or car, or when screwing in a wood screw or on your wheel nuts maybe. It is great for anything that needs lubricating a little without staining then dries up, but it is not for internal use.
It will one day have a label on the bottle "DO NOT INGEST".
Until then, consider it has that label.

With the continuing degeneration of people's health there manifests another benefit for the pharmaceutical or chemical industry. The production of even more toxic substance that are prescribed to you by your doctor. These however only disguise the symptoms (yes, they just disguise the symptoms) of whatever you are suffering from. Not one actually fixes the problem or attempts to get to the core of the issue.   And what is more, they have a myriad of direct and detrimental effects as stated earlier strangely called side affects. How is an affect a side affect when it is caused directly from taking the substance. You don't say the effects of drinking alcohol has the side affect of getting drunk, it is rubbish, nonsense, idiotic, ridiculous and may I add, just more deception.
With the knowledge available, these chemicals prescribed by doctors, could sometimes be made to actually help or even bring some degree of cure to some of the issues you face. Instead they only help you to feel a little better for a while. Unless they can justify high prices and continuous consumption there is no money in it. This would not make economic sense to the pharmaceutical companies. To produce a cure may make them 100 £ounds, $ollars, €uros, where as a product to only disguise the symptoms will mean you need it for life and will make them tens of thousands and sometimes millions and even billions of £ounds, $ollars and €uros or whatever other made up currency you can think of.
You must see that this is not the answer to your health issues.

This leads on to another problem of Doctors education once out in their practices.
When my friends entered the medical profession, they all had high hopes of being able to help people and most of them still do even though their actions may be questionable.

Why is that?
Well it all comes from their ongoing education and whom it comes from. You see once medical school is over, which incidentally is designed and focused to support big Pharma and their medical model, the only education of new ideas and practices that come to the doctor are from a Drug salesperson. There is little time in their money-making program even to read the medical journal's that are often delivered to their practice. What the drug salesperson brings and also contributes to their income and there may even be a new jaguar or holiday for the family as an added incentive if they can promote/prescribe enough of it.

Is it any wonder that doctors are way behind the rest of us in recognizing issues, just like my old doctor was when he said "Fatigue is only in the head so I will send you to a psychiatrist." Even worse, is when you explain something, they will ignore you with a look of "I know best so stop wasting my time."
It happens to take ten or more years of suffering themselves before doctors start recognizing what you and I see to be true today.

Thought: Why is it when you go to the doctor you have to go to their place of practice. Because they are not sure what the hell they are doing and really are only "practicing", on you.

As if this wasn't enough for the greed of the chemical industry they have since try to capture and control world food supplies through genetic modifying as many foods as they can Patent….
Should they ever succeed in getting control of this, the world would slip into starvation very quickly as they could never produce enough seed to feed the world's population. Perhaps this is already happening and why their need for vaccines to control unrest, or worst kill off the population as and when they see fit.

In this book we have not even taken into account any other possible effects as yet largely unknown to you other than the compromise of your gut and immune system at this time by eating strangely modified produce that are totally unnecessary other than for control and profit.

- None of the GMO's are about feeding the world.

- They are about controlling food supplies.

Note: It would be wise for you to keep in mind that you are at the end of the food chain and that whatever they tamper with or alter unnaturally today will most certainly have its effect on you at some time in the near future.

The food pyramid.

The next major consideration to think about is the food pyramid. Was it good intention or blatant manipulation of misinformation, and influence by the producers when developing the food pyramid?
We can only guess, but whatever the intention the end results have been catastrophic as the major emphasis is on eating refined carbohydrate. Whether this was intentional or not it all flows along the same lie we have been led down since the 1930's.

The very things you should be avoiding or at least eating very little of, is the base and the biggest aspect of this idea.
 It is clear now that it was designed for profit, not health.

THE ORIGINAL FOOD PYRAMID

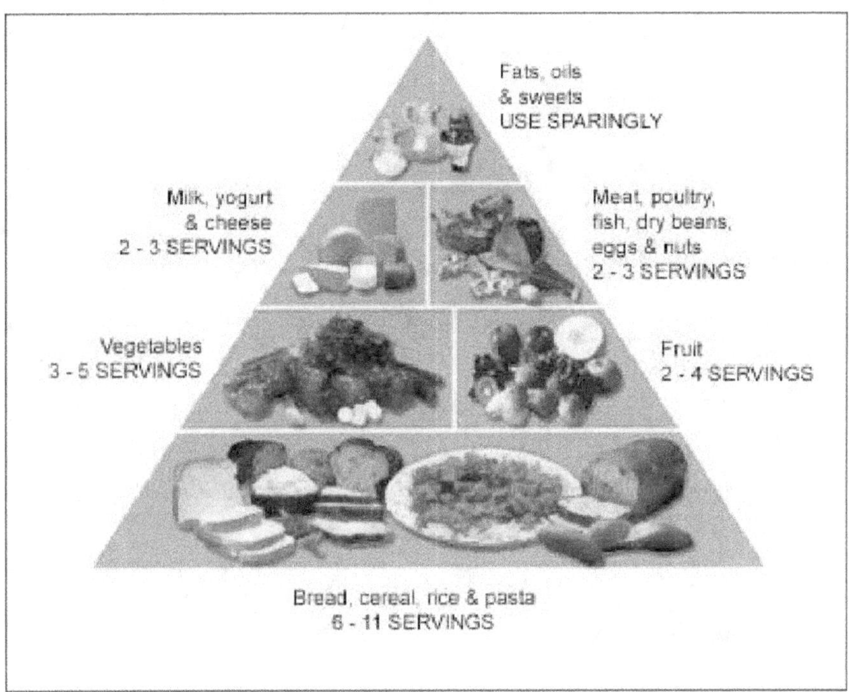

Superimpose another pyramid on top upside down and what is in the middle of the 2 pyramids would be somewhat better.

I would call this the food diamond and I recommend you consider looking at this and using the proportions within the new diamond area as it is shown below:

We have done it for you,

The Health Whispers
BETTER FOOD GUIDE;

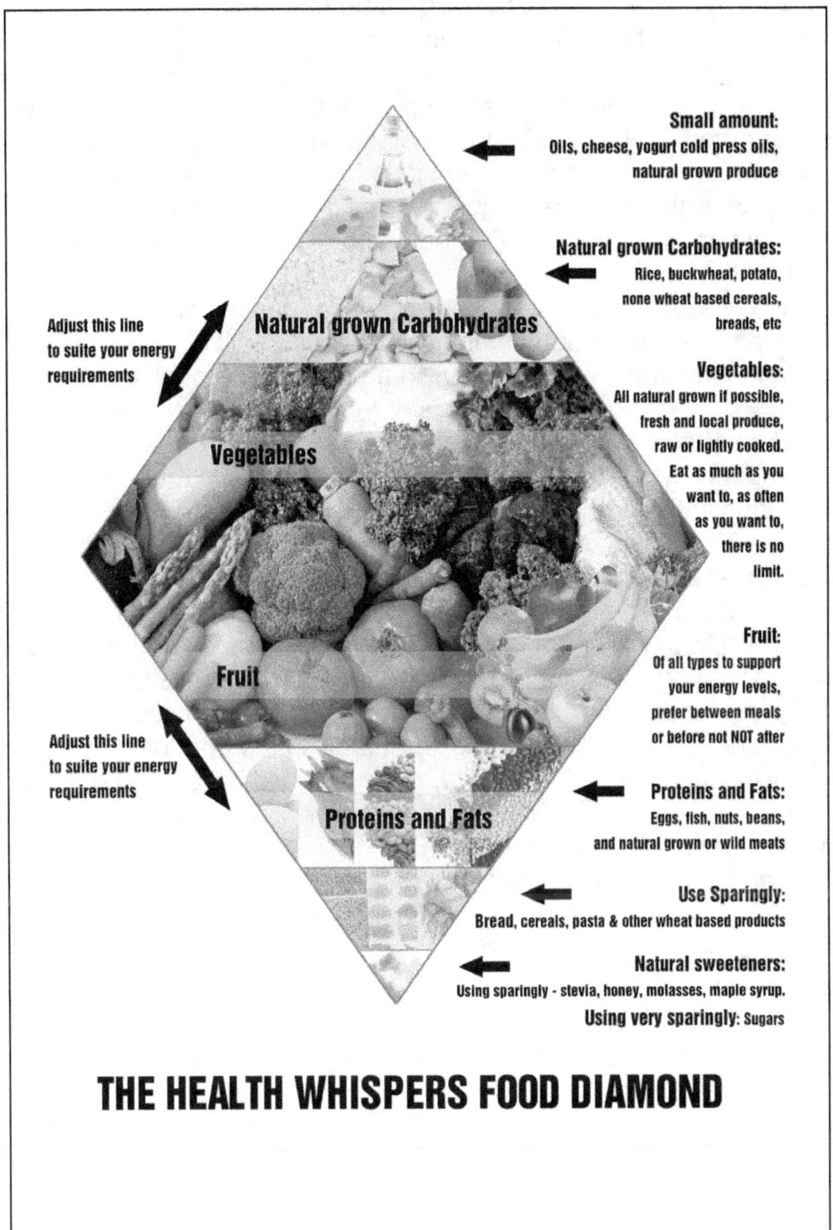

THE HEALTH WHISPERS FOOD DIAMOND

BETTER FOOD GUIDE

Remember
The Health Whispers **Better Food Guide is just a GUIDE** to help
you find the food balance best for you

I hope you are starting to get the picture that at least 75% or more
of your food intake is to be fresh vegetables and some fruits,
preferably without modern chemicals (as you can eat as much as
you want without concern) and the rest of your food intake to be of
natural carbohydrate, proteins and some fruit with only a very little
of the other stuff if you must.
You may also note, there is no processed food acceptable other
than in very small amounts unless you preserve it or mess it up
yourself and know what's in it. And no need for calorie counting.

Back to History
The next Huge lie that started in the early 1970's is the low-fat diet.
This was initially devised from a student doing a thesis on feeding
fat to rabbits. The study should be questioned anyway just for the
idea of fat being feed to rabbits is ridiculous.
He found when he did his autopsy on the rabbits that their arteries
were blocked with fatty deposits. This is all very well and good for
rabbits, but humans are not rabbits. Rabbits have evolved to only
eat grass and other vegetation not fat. This study however is very
inconclusive as we are not told what fat was fed and for all we
know it could have been veg-oil and this would have proved there
and then not to use it. Whichever it was we were all misled by the
twist of the information, again for profit.
Human evolution is very different, we require some fats for the
benefit of body muscle, brain and heart function. Without these
building blocks, our bodies do not function very well at all and may
eventually shut down.

If FAT really was the problem, then the Eskimos
would be long dead or even extinct
as they traditionally live on fat and a little meat
for most of the year even today.

This low fat fad was, and still is another wonderful opener to create
huge profits for the food industry and then the pharmaceutical

industry and has turned a stupid idea into a multi-billion dollar business selling virtual waste products to the consumer then pretending to fix the health issues with further toxic chemicals by way of this pill or that pill or even worse the sharp knife of exploration surgery.

Note the word exploration. Doctors have no more clue than the rest of us what they will find when they do surgery, that's why they think they need to hack into people just to explore or experiment to see if they can work out something. When they cannot work out what to label it, they make it up.

No I did not make that up, normal human thinking could not make up such a destructive system, but it is what happens and it is all about money not health

.

Take away the fat and most of what's left is lifeless dead waste, and to make it taste of anything resembling food it is loaded with excessive amounts of salt, sugar, preservatives, and other chemicals. They have to lace them with these substances, or you would not eat them. Without them you would probably prefer to eat the cardboard or paper packaging or even suck on a plastic bag. And because they are laced with these substances, especially sugar and salt, they become extremely addictive and you go back and back and back for more and more of this so-called food that is starving you at best and more likely poisoning you too.

In the past few years there is more and more information and research being published on the effects of sugar. The most frustrating thing of all is that the research was done some 30 or so years ago on what really was the cause of the obesity and many other health issues.

An English man called John S. YUDKIN had the information correct in his report/book "Pure White and Deadly" written in the 1970's but was discredited in America by way of the low fat program with their eyes on the money for the food industry. And more recently On May 26, 2009, Robert Lustig gave a lecture called "Sugar: The Bitter Truth," that was in the NY times and then published on YouTube. Check them out for yourself if they have not been taken down.

Following close on the heels of the low-Fat scam and probably the best of all cons of the food industry, is to increase of the size of the portions of those virtual waste products mentioned above. The sizing has increased to what is now called super-size.

Double the size of pop for example and they treble or more their profits from all sides.

You may note that as the sizing has increased (in all the places subject to the over sizing abuse on us all) so has the very same super sizing reality of obesity manifested itself in the humanity that frequents those same joints.

Look at what size you are
then look at what you eat,
there is a direct connection.

It is clear that the food industry has made even more $billions from this "Super Sizing" idea alone while you suffer not just the dead and waste foods dished up to you in a nose bag everywhere you go now, but you are now faced with mountains more of it than your body can possibly handle. But you stuff it in, in the hope of some value that's not there.

When we check back in time to the 70's and before we find that there were few places to get so called fast food and people would go out for a treat maybe once a week at best for a burger at the local tuck shop (takeaway place). A burger (one) made of real meat in an almost real bun was all they would have with lots of salad on the side and a cup of tea or maybe a small pop if available (approx. 7 oz or 200 mils) not even a ¼ litre.

Now it's a meal deal in a nose bag
of Air bun, Slime burger, Fries,
and 2 Litres of refillable Pop.

In the example here, the dead foods are bad enough and very addictive, but the Pop is the real killer with almost 50 teaspoons of a deadly toxin and slow killer called sugar. It's enough toxin in one dose to turn a fully grown elephant cross eyed and make its knees weak and wobbly, but you pour it down your throat several times a day and don't expect any harm to come to you.

It is pure crazy thinking and Einstein's version of insanity.

Are you really that gullible or even that stupid?
Not to see this as it is and just accept what they say as true
or have you been blind folded and brainwashed
by their lies in pursuit of profit
look up, open your eyes, and start to live again

Perhaps it is not all your fault, as you have been misled by and for
the benefit of the big corporations. They have taken responsibility
to make money for their shareholders but not to be responsible with
what they promote to you to achieve it or your health.

It may NOT be all, your fault,
because you have been misled.
However, the responsibility,
still remains with YOU and each one of us
 to inform yourself and act on it correctly.

Will you reconsider your position and decide whether you wish to
continue supporting these big corporations at the expense of your
own health and wealth too?
Or take responsibility for yourself and simply stop eating their slime,
waste and poisons.

The big corporations have not taken their part in being responsible
to you at all, the truth is they do not care about you, only their
bottom line (money) and have reached the levels of legalise fraud
to achieve it so you are tasked with taking your own responsible
action to consider your own health, your own wealth.

Yes, It is time for you to take responsibility for yourself.
Start by Just walking past their door but never through it.
Start by supporting your local farm suppliers first.
Start by setting up local and community grow projects.
Start by only buying the whole and nature's own, grown produce

Please Note that All of the above is Just an introduction to get you
started thinking so you will understand a least a little about the
importance of what you do. YOU really do make a difference.

Taking it even Further
These next few realities are interesting to consider.

Should you trust the US Food and drug administration (FDA)
While recently in America there was much talk of Gun control.
There are some 16,000, gun related deaths every year in America,
half of which are killed by cops. Yes that's right killed by over force
of the law by the very same cops you mistakenly think are there to
protect you.
And about 11,000 suicide's which many are related to the gun.
A sure sign that the gun is not actually the problem, but the mental
state of the nation is. It's all about how the people and yes that's
you, are coerced, controlled and suppressed by the dependable's
to benefit big corporate profits and shadow control.
 Where has the hope gone?

This, however sad and tragic as the gun deaths are, it is just
another welcome distraction and in reality, small change when
compared to the real issues that are so often hidden for you or
quashed by the official line: -
Pharmaceuticals drugs are known to kill more than 225,000 people
every year in the USA alone and it is estimated that this number is
actually more than 785,000 per year who die unnecessarily for the
greed of others in pushing their toxic but legalised crap.
If you relay these numbers throughout the world the present
medical complex is killing millions of people every year through
their legalised, inadequate and toxic methods, all in the name of
profit.
Its legalised murder that MUST STOP.

Are officials deceiving the people to protect an industry.
Listen carefully to the media and you will get snippets of scandal
after scandal regarding the inappropriate actions of the
Pharmaceutical and Food industries from bad practice and bad
drugs to bribing officials and doctors. Whatever scam they think
they can get away with in their march for money they have already
tried and will again try it on, even to killing those that speak out
against their practices and misinformation. They have even got
laws enacted for you to pay for any law suit against them through
government pay-outs. Their favourite story line when someone

speaks out about their bad practices is that it is just a conspiracy theory and what they are doing is good. I ask you to see through this line and understand it is only good for them, not you.

There are more than 60 thousand manufactured chemicals flowing around in the system we live in and that we are subjected to daily. Yes, you read that right more than 60,000 manufactured chemicals, in fact it is estimated to be more likely to be closer to 100,000. The real problem is not only that these manufactured chemicals are being produced but that only a very small fraction of them have ever undergone any real testing regarding their safety to human health yet all are known to affect your health in some way even to death. In spite of these facts the FDA turn a blind eye to them and pretend all is well until something very serious happens.

Only when it is proved that many people have been severely affected will they drag their feet, sidestep or just pretend to look into the problem. Then it mysteriously just disappears, and nothing is done so big business can carry on as usual greasing their palms. Take and consider just one of these manufactured chemicals, the Opioid pain killers, kill almost 100,000 people every year in the USA alone and many thousands more around the world. This is on top of the other numbers mentioned above. Its murder for profit. This is More deaths than can be associated to ALL the so call illegal drugs combined from just one so called pain killer. Perhaps they should be called the "Killer" drug (along with all the others) or can you add the word "Pain" in there. Perhaps the word pain can be added as once you're dead there will be no more physical pain at least for you but it's extremely selfish as there will be a lot of pain for those who loved you.

Aside from the deaths that occur each year due to pharmaceutical poisoning and error, there are many thousands of people with their bodies shut down or severely compromised. This is especially true of the older folks today as they have been conditioned to believe in their doctors as if they are gods, the all wise, all knowing god. Whatever they say must be true and also must be followed. This belief is literally killing our older generation, slowly and painfully, leaving them without any quality of life, often for many years. Some I know spent the last 20 plus years in a semi vegetative state while their bodies hung on to life. This is no way to treat your enemy let alone your mum and dad.

Also think about the actual reasons why most people visit the chemist. Cold & Flu? Pain Relief? Fertility Problems? Weight Loss? High Cholesterol? Nutritional Deficiencies? and so on. In most cases these frequent issues can be easily corrected with maintaining a healthy lifestyle and eating correctly (provided the food you eat has nutritional value).

> Rather than masking the problem with drugs
> it is better to address and treat the problem at its core.

Now there is a novel idea, an idea that used to be before the modern medical model pushed them all out so they could win.

When you stop and think about it, it seems a lot insane to guzzle down a cocktail of chemical drugs (pills) to reduce or disguise the effects from your very own poor lifestyle choices.

Don't be fooled into thinking that an industry
that relies on your sickness
to make billions of dollars each year
really wants you to have good health.
We say
Why not just make your health a choice instead?
An industry that truly cared for your health
would teach you to adapt lifestyle habits
that support lasting health and longevity
not the taking of yet more toxins for them to profit from.

So why does the FDA in all its alleged wisdom continue condoning and legitimizing all these known to be toxic agricultural chemicals, drugs and poisons as they do?
The answer is simple. They have a policy of employment exchange with the big boys. You will find if you only look a little, that the people in the FDA have either worked with in the past or are going to work for a pharmaceutical or agricultural company once they leave the FDA position. It is therefore, all about protecting THEIR interest and THEIR future, not yours.

It's up to you to take control of your own health

That is, if you want it to be good.

Should we trust the US Department of agriculture (USDA) and their guidelines.

Is this Yet another action of officials deceiving the people to protect an industry. This department is the same as the FDA with its revolving door of exchange employment.

In January 2011 The Department of Agriculture announced the release of the 2010 Dietary guidelines For Americans," the federal government's evidence-based nutritional guidance to promote health reduce the risk of chronic diseases, and reduce the prevalence of overweight and obesity through improved nutrition and physical activity."

 If only it were true.

It is interesting to note that for some 30 years now the doctor's guidelines for America have been recommending an increase in carbohydrate consumption and a decrease in saturated fat and animal protein.

In the same time frame the result of these recommendations, Overweight, obesity, and diabetes have increased to epidemic proportions.

The 2010 Dietary guidelines further increase the recommendations for carbohydrate intake and further decrease its recommendation for saturated fat and animal protein.

Even worse they recommend starting these Recommendations with children from birth. This means that children will be deprived of the very nutrients that are critical for the development of their brain, which affect not only their thinking ability but also behaviour and mood stabilization. These nutrients, which include: Vegetables, fruit, Essential Fatty acids (EFA's) and cholesterol which are found in, or assimilated from, animal fats, eggs, fish, nuts and seeds, all of which were recommended to be restricted.

While they are recommending trans fats like margarine, Crisco and vegetable oils which are known to cause inflammation, depress the immune system, lead to cancer and more significantly directly related to heart dis-ease and stroke. Why because they make Money by the billions from your sickness.

So the answer here is NO as with the FDA as it is clear who's field they are standing in.

There are other reasons why this line is continuing and you only have to look at "agenda 21" and "2030", "event 201" and others but do your own research on this. You may be shocked if and when you truly understand the truth behind these programs.

Lets get back to what is affecting you right now.

Whereas the benefits to you are amazing, of natural and animal fats for growth, immunity, neurological function and general body and bone health. You stay healthy, so for them No Money from your sickness.

Even in the journal "Nutrition" They state important aspects of these recommendations remain unproven and recommend returning to an evidence-based methodology.

It is clear that the new USDA guidelines are set out for the benefit of big business and industry addicted to profits and not for the People's benefit or better health, reduced weight and well-being.

What about the CIA, can they be trusted?

You may believe that the CIA was set up as an intelligence agency to keep the people of America safe, well you would be wrong. The interesting thing though is that it runs on your tax money but It was set up to manipulate the world for the benefit of the shadow controllers and money manipulators who now own or control some 90% of all big companies around the world. Bought by the CIA operatives on their behalf I might add and sometimes way over their real value just to get hold of the control. Not to worry though about paying over the odds as they just make up the money on a computer so who cares what it costs and anyway, they have politicians in their pockets to bail them out with your backing if it all goes down. Another interesting point related to this is that some 40% of these companies are running at a loss while you are incentivised to invest in them to keep them running for the excess to be bled off the top before they finally crash in your lap.

The cia is yet another extension of government used as an instrument against the people of the world, especially the poor and mostly paid for by the poor in their unlawful taxes

The **UN and WHO** are no better, set up by the controllers for you pay while they control you into accepting the new world order.

How far will these institutions go to control you and erase your freedom, your status and even your life. Speak the truth on anything that does not hold their narrative and you will see. They will assassinate your character and even take your life to keep their lies and fraud in line with their desire for power. Already they have surveillance on you beyond your imagination and you have told them everything about yourself already on fb and google, Instagram and twitter. The reality is the game they play is finite and played for them to win and only them to win. Whereas life is infinite and better played for everyone to win so we can all keep playing. Maybe it is important to add here that the WHO, world health organisation and the UN, united nations were also set up to push the goals of the shadow controllers and not to help the world.

These are all sad stories of deceit and greed I know but they need to be told. Unfortunately, what you read here is just the tip of their iceberg of the misinformation put out today. I just give you an overview because you cannot unknow something once you already know it and sometimes it is better to know just enough to understand why there must be other and better ways for humanity.

> All is not lost and there is something you can do.
> When you care about life,
> nature, the environment and the future
> you must have censorship resistance
> and look through their smoke screen.
> Question everything as all is not as it seems.

Question, Question, Question everything. Start with what you believe first of all then what you are told, by any so called professional or expert as you are most likely being told only their truth for their benefit. When you complete their story you may be surprised to find it's their agenda staring back at you and its almost certainly not of any real benefit to you.

Socialism

There is a massive move toward the left and socialism today with the popular concept of more equality. In principal this all sounds great but who exactly is behind it and what is true.

Who's STORY is it anyway as stated earlier?
Beware because it is the story put out by the 1%, the super-rich
and there is a very good reason they want you to think socialism is
for you and that is because it is for them. Socialism is the absolute
and ultimate form of capitalism for those in control as they get all
the money, power and control to play with, while you get all the
work and pain to do, to get it for them. And because they have all
the power and control over you history shows it very quickly turns
to fascism and disaster for the masses. E.g. Starlin, Moa and Hitler.
It is fool's gold, full of lies and empty promises and must be
avoided and a search for better ways to live embarked upon.
Also be watchful of any ism for what and who is behind the story.
You just have to look at the last few major experiments with isms to
see just how dangerous it is for humanity. The ideology sounds
great to the loving human mind but it is far from it and once you
give them even a shadow of agreement they seize power and take
you through the gates of hell. Take the socialist experiment of
communism in china with a 100 million people dead in the initial
transition and destruction of their society and still the atrocities are
ongoing today. Then there is the Russian, USSR experiment where
just under Stalin more than 30 million were sent to Siberia never to
return, all dead and many millions more starved to death when the
food they grew was taken from them for the elites. And what about
Nazi-ism where the death toll is again unimaginable and could
again be around 100 million or more. And then there are the wars
all around the world that have followed WW2 under elite-ism where
many hundreds of millions more have either been killed or their
lives destroyed and the rest of us are in despair in the name of their
profiteering and greed. You only need to look at Yemen, Iraq and
Syria today to see what they have planned for you and your family
too. Yes, it is so important to reject all such ism's for they all end in
disaster for humanity.

Individual and nation sovereignty
working in unity and cooperation together for a better way
to lift our human capital to fulfil our true potential
would be a good starting point
No special interest lobbyists allowed

I know I go on about the Shadow Controllers a lot in this book, but it is so important to understand what is happening and where we are today because not only your health but your freedoms too are so severely affected by their actions. Surely you must see it now for it is manifesting all around you right now.

They already own and control almost everything.
They own and control the MSMedia, that is everything you see on TV, the news, the movie industry, they own and control the UN and WHO, most governments around the world, all of which you pay for, the money system and supply, 90% of all big Corporations bought up with their fake money and worst of all they have control over the so called secret service and legal systems of so many countries especially the cia, the fbi and even worse the teacher training and Education system in most countries to twist the minds of your young and now they are in the last faze to literally own and control everything.
That means your house, your car, your business, your life and yes that means you and your children too.

Will you wait till there is nothing left to live for before you do anything to stop them?

These are the same group of controllers behind communism in Russia and china, Nazi-ism and all the wars and major atrocity's over the past hundred years and more at least that they say is about religion or communism, all the unrest wherever it has taken place to todays, black lives matter, anti Semitism and every other unrest activity you can think of although some are good causes to support they are hijacked and paid for by the left. Each one created for them to gain yet another power position in their quest for total control.
Almost all politicians but the Left in politics is especially controlled by these evil money men and do not be fooled by all their nice talk of a better world, they are hollow words for you because you are in their way of a better world for them and their intention is that you will be eradicated so they can have their better world.
In fact left leaning politics and its followers for all their talk of a better world seem now to be based on hearsay, hypocrisy, filled hatred hell bent on revenge on everything and everyone that shows

any sign of questioning their hate fill narrative. Look closely and you will see through their talk for their actions show exactly what they plan and their reverse speak is filled with hate. They are the ones destroying the cities, burning buildings, rioting, destroying all possibility of you being able to earn a living and support your family and burning the crops so you cannot eat. They are the ones that twist the truth, so you and I think we are enemy's and fight each other while they laugh out loud and seize power over us all. These are all the things Hitler did to gain power and I say to you beware for it is the beginnings of their final phase to fascism. If history is our guide they are all ism's to be avoided for they have always turned to tyranny.

Don't get me wrong there are plenty of politicians on all sides that have no integrity and were willing to do things that compromise themselves and now they are controlled by these money men's blackmail. That is why you must be vigilant and only support the ones that are there to serve you with integrity.

We are at the gates of hell once again
don't be fooled by the left-ism talk of a better world,
for it is just propaganda to get you to agree
for them to open the gates
and lead you into hell one last time.

This is their final goal to own and control everything and if we do not stand against this now together with everyone else, they really will create Hell for humanity right here on this beautiful earth.
Until you are aware of this and openly reject it with conscious thought and a clear statement there is no way for humanity to be safe from their dark ideas and controls.
When you do, you shine your light on them and as they only function in darkness this removes their power over you. The more of us that do this the less power they have to make our lives the Hell they plan.

Your action is important and needed NOW
Start by casting your vote for humanity and truth.
Decide carefully.

10 EDUCATE

Remember it is the left generally the shadow controllers have control over because that is the best system for them to create total power over you when they are done but watch quietly and you will see and hear the talk of the controlled ones for it is not of love for humanity. There are so many in all political parties that have been bribed and compromised and now controlled against you so think from your heart for whom to vote for then demand they serve you. Or better still stand yourself as an independent so that these compromised ones are shown for what they are.
We need you now.

Can we?

Can we create a better future?
From the corporate and governmental tyranny against us
And their destructive desires
in the same boxed thinking that created today
NO
Some will say it can't be done
Others will find a way and reasons why it can
Step outside the boxes of past constraints
Open your hearts and minds
To new and inspiring knowledge
Available to you now
Take the action
Working on it together
Yes we can

Living in compassion for others
For the human next to you is not the enemy
The controlling reptilians' are
Humans my friends, come together
Unite, all as one
To create and build a better way
In the human freedom
Of spirit love
Reconnect to your purpose
No harm to others
No approval necessary
Do what you can today
To ensure tomorrow a better place

11 CUTTING EDGE

Rethink, For a future that may just work

We are energetic beings
Unfortunately, so much of what is done
by the controllers of today
stalls your potential
now that we are stopped let us clear this stupidity
and work within nature as intended
to regain the natural gifts of energy
of life.

There is way too much important information to improve things for one Rethink, but I will give you a few ideas to start thinking about Remember that thinking and doing the same tomorrow as you do today will just get you the same old shit, if that is your status quo…

Rethinking today is more important than ever because the last rethink on the social conscious and structure of things was not a rethink that has worked for you and me or any of the people's around the world. Just take note of the unhappy people in so many countries today. It has pretended to keep us free from troubles and pain but there is no freedom to do anything for ourselves. The stage is set to keep maintaining the balance in "favour of the few" they are creating more and more troubles and pain by way of controls and restrictions like forced taxes, vaccinations, environmental blame and wherever you look you are being controlled, coerced and forced to do things you probably would not do if your mind was free to choose, and therefore you are so brainwashed or controlled that you do them seeming willingly.
We are all so close to being under water, figuratively steaking, that it is a wonder that any of us can breath at all. Gasping for air.

What will you do when things are not by the rule of law
And you are ruled by fear?
Take a stand while it is still possible
Take back control
Your voice and vote matters
Sovereignty and freedom for all

The first step in any Rethink is to find and understand the truth of things and the way to do this is to question everything, absolutely everything starting with your own beliefs.

Ask
1. What are they, my beliefs, where did they come from and do they serve me?
2. What is being said and what are the facts about this, and do they make sense especially when alongside other information?
3. Who is saying it, and what do they gain from it?
4. Who is behind them i.e. who's drum are they banging and what do those people gain from it?
5. Does the story improve my life and help me get to my desired place, goal, weight, or whatever my outcome is?
6. Is there love, respect and compassion in what is being said
7. Does this or can this work and benefit all of humanity?

You may need to add your own questions too

When you ask questions like these then you see that much of what you are told today is not for your benefit, and is certainly not the truth in any way for humanity.

The Rethink

Once we have all come together to remove the power and money of the controllers by quietly removing our support and loudly stating that what they are doing we do not agree too and must stop now. Then we can get onto creating a different and better future.

Let's start with Farmers as they are the life blood of your existence for without them you will not have food to eat. Support the farmers that are open to production with natural, sustainable methods that actually protect our earth and are working within nature's own system. If they do not, then walk past their door too, for without this change there is no benefit to your health or humanity as a whole.

 And what about the good stuff that was banned and restricted from the people, all the people of the world.

Marijuana and Hemp

There are many plants that have amazing and magical healing properties for so many different issues but when the research on this range of plants is observed, as there are many, the properties and multiple uses it can be applied to, and the significant benefits to humanity are understood, then you can only call them the wonder plants.
They can be made into a range of the best rope, sacking, towelling, clothing all the way through to the other end of the scale where it offers many very important healing and health properties, health benefits and pain reducing abilities. There may also be further benefits to calming your chatter in your head and getting you closer to the place of deep velvet quiet of the awake brain, your spiritual guide and mentor. Today it is forbidden you connect with that as you may start thinking for yourself. The evil controllers would not want that.
Most of the real benefits come not from smoking it as most people in this banned situation seem to want to do but from the consumption of the oil through evaporation and eating the leaves and buds throughout its growth. All of us should have a few plants in our garden for health just like we grow herbs for health.
Keep that quiet too or they will ban herbs next

But it was banned and every effort was made to hide it from the people just like all the other great things that have come for the people throughout the last 100 years or so but they too were banned or stolen and hidden and the inventors killed so the controllers controlled the supply, the resources and made all the money.

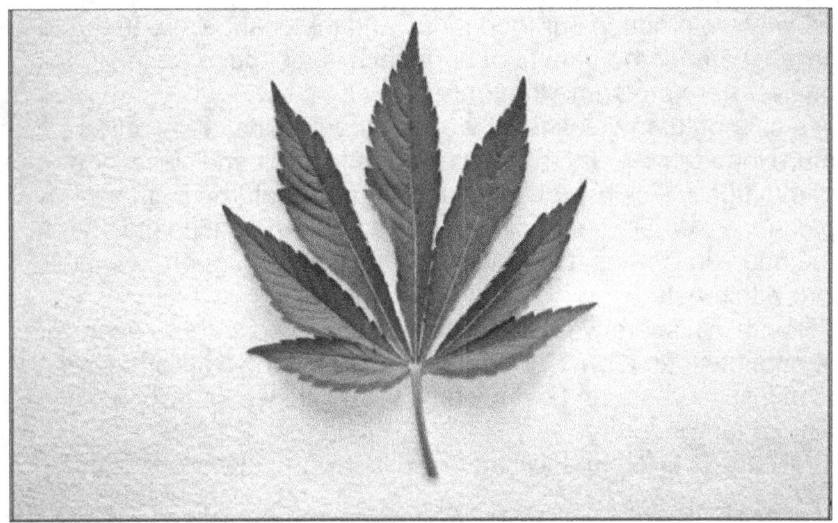

So why was it banned and given such a bad rap –

At the early part of last century, (1900's) this range of plants were observed to be wonder plants of many uses. Unfortunately, it was considered of great competition to other industries. Those industries, the cotton growers, the oil and chemical industries, were not prepared to stand by and risk losing some of their own markets to it. Perhaps they were right to be afraid of the lose of business because of the truly wonderous properties within the full range of these plants

They lobbied congress (of course this happened in America, where else, where all the politicians are buyable) with much pressure and millions of dollars to manipulate the politicians to have this threat stopped. The government responded with having all of it, yes that is the whole range of plants in the family, banned and made the laws to make them all illegal to grow, hold or possess.

Of course this was not enough to just have this ridiculous law to themselves, so like so many other draconian control mechanism's forced on the rest of the world before and since, by the US government this one too was forced on the rest of the world.

Now we live in the shadow of force against it on the one side and knowing the loss of benefit, just out of reach, on the other.

The Production of Food

The way we produce our food today and the change's required to correct them for the benefit of our health is too much for this book however here are some thoughts.

"We cannot keep doing what we have been doing and control nature long term, or try to dominate or change it artificially, nature will eventually kick back against us. Against natures Roth we have no chance". What chance do you have surviving a tsunami if you are caught in it, almost zero without mysterious support, we must work within nature,

At Health Whispers we have observed this to be so true, even with the changes of the past 70 years or so. Let alone what's happened in the last 10 years and even worse what little we know of what is planned for the future.

REMEMBER --- Nature will have the last word, always……

Young people, pick up the cause,
relearn the old technic's of caring for and feeding the soil,
and make, or force the changes back to nature's own.
in the future you will say
what were our forbearers doing
In hate and war, control and coercion, suppression and greed
while farming and health were based on poisons
what on this good earth were they thinking?
I will tell you
they were sleep walking.

What can you do?

Start by doing some of you own searching and develop your own Resource section for you to refer to

Check out   HealthWhispers.com/Articles
for some initial reading to start your search and find other sources too.

Get together in your neighbourhood with as many as possible and cultivate every bit of ground you can find to grow vegetables. Start on your own if you have to and soon others will want to join in.

Doing this enables you, together with your neighbours (if done properly) to get back to locally grown food. Grown with nature and nurture without chemicals and sharing the love of nature together. It also creates a local and supportive community where everyone is willing to help and watch out for each other. Not only will you all be eating better food but when done ethically you will all also benefit from the human connection, the way we are designed to connect and support each other

This example is a great place to aim to start from, wherever you are in the world

Stop buying the crap and start growing your own real food.

Farming and the production of food

When farming is considered properly whatever the focus of production the first place to start, is to farm the water. Without the water nothing grows and when water is present things grow and the water comes even more. Just like your gut and brain work together so do most things in nature. One and all together in nature makes perfect while humans seem to desire to separate to concur which sadly ends in destruction of the land and shortage of food. Then there is the growing of crops including vegetation for the animals, the soils must be replenished and feed for that which is grown to be healthy and nutrient rich.

When domestic animals are part of the plan, they must be roamed (preferably with predators or predator like actions) as in nature. When this is done correctly and without the modern chemicals, the animals are healthy, the environment recovers, even the deserts will recover, and the water will return to the land and therefore more can be produced. Animals in nature eating the food they were designed to eat do not produce all the methane that grain feed animals do so there is another win situation there for you environmentalists.

There is such fear instilled in all of you these days that you cannot even see the possibility of these change's let alone the benefits to the land, the farmer and the environment as a whole. And farmers are so protective of their animals they kill the predators but the loss of the odd animal to a predator is a small price to pay for the bigger benefit of having the predator around for better farming.

Predators should be reintroduced and welcomed and where there were no predators create a system or scenario to mimic their presence. This is to stir up the animals and loosen the soils to make it more porous so that water can enter, and it works like magic when the next rains come.

In most cases due to the benefits of having the predators around more stock could be run on the land because the land recovers and the green recovers. Once balance with nature is achieved everything grows to achieve its balance too but this time in a healthy way. When working in nature the vegetation will support much more of everything. All of this applies to growing food too when the soils are replenished with nature much more will grow and there are many trials that have proved this but this info does not come out or is squashed by big business control.

My Dad talked of "**Farming with Nature**" when I was nursing him in the last months of his life as he realised the terrible mistakes of contaminating the soils with modern chemical methods, his health for one is a major indicator of the stupidity of the use of farming with toxic chemicals. The same applies to thousands of farmers around the world that use these methods.

I first saw the practice of natural farming which starts with farming water in Africa where green vegetation grew all year round, surrounded by dry baron lands. I have since come across it in Australia, the Americas, South east Asia and other places too where enlightened people understand the importance of working with nature and not controlling, resisting or forcing it. I have seen this first-hand, but you can see for yourself as there are now many videos on YouTube and elsewhere that show these things in action. It is truly amazing the difference farming the water and working in nature makes.

Why we went down the other route of intensive, chemical filled farming was mis information projected only for the profit of big Pharma while their lust for greed sees more and more controls and manipulation taking place today, physical, financial and genetic, i.e. GMO. Had farmers followed the cycles and systems of nature as they had for thousands of years we would have far more food than the world needs today to feed the people and the food would be of nature, that means, have value and be full of nutrition.

There is also the issue with supermarkets and their desire for form, this form is in the guise of the perfect shape to sell. Nature does not work that way and today some 48% or more of all food produced in the western world is discarded because it does not "look" right. Stupidity at its best.

Then there is the use of natural mineral fertilisers from both sea and land, discussed within to replenish the soil and not toxify it.

There is so much more to working with in nature for this book.

Some other thoughts for you.

Climate Change
What is Climate change and are you really the cause?
There is much that we all must do better in support of our planet, like protecting its lungs and life, Forests and Oceans, not polluting it with plastic, waste and toxic chemicals, or destroying the biodiversity and killing the animals and so much more.

However it is a very strange issue at this time, the subject of global warming now changed to be called climate change. This in itself should raise the red flags of inconsistency. It is a hot topic and so many activists seem to be sold out on the subject yet so out of touch with the facts. If you question what is put forward by them they do not seem to have any real answers and just rant dogma at you. You know there is no substance in their story when critique is just rejected by discrediting and slandering the assessor.
One thing that seems to be lost on them is the fact that the projected thinking/outcome is based on the last 300 to 400 years. The strange thing is that the earth has been around for billions of years so the first question to ask is how does the last 400 years relate to the several billion years of the earths existence.

And if you look over the ice core samples and geological observations for the last billion years or so the earth has survived much higher temperatures and significantly higher levels of carbon dioxide so what in fact is the real issue. It is also interesting to note that carbon levels do not go along with temperature trends on the historical analyses, there is no constant correlation. Even the last ten thousand years shows many peaks and troughs similar to the last 300 years rise to today's temperatures, yet carbon levels have continued reducing throughout this time. The one issue that really does not make sense is the cry to be carbon neutral. This one important fact of getting carbon neutral seems to be lost in all the frenzy to work toward reducing carbon dioxide emissions. Well if you study the geological observations of carbon dioxide you will learn that the levels of carbon dioxide are possibly at the lowest level in the atmosphere in the last million years or so at least. If this geological analysis is correct and there is no reason to dispute it, it would mean that putting some carbon dioxide back into the atmosphere should be a good thing. Not according to the outspoken on the subject. My Question is, what is the real intention of the money people (the controllers) who started the movement. Is it the reduction and starvation of humanity so they have better control over the population while they pump their own greenhouses full of carbon dioxide to grow their food? This practice already happens today in greenhouse growing because of the extremely low levels of it in the atmosphere. Carbon dioxide is the very thing plants take in to grow, then they do a magical thing and turn out oxygen in return. It's a beautiful cyclical process in a very delicate balance for survival of life.

If we do not do it, the earth will have to re-balance the levels itself by erupting in volcanic activity. As you may note it has begun to do in recent years, after a long and reasonably quiet period. There is a line with nature, and it balances itself just nicely around this line without our interference or panic about it doing so.

The real issue that they have caused by all this toxic activity but it is never mentioned and that is the reduction of oxygen to the lowest levels for life just like the carbon levels for plants human and animal life is in danger from lack of oxygen too. They have cut down the lungs of the planet, the forests to feed you McDonald's and you stuff them down your neck as if nothing is wrong and polluted the oceans too, that produce the oxygen.

The planet may exist but life on it may not if this stupidity continues.

11 CUTTING EDGE

Now all of the talk out there is that we are all to blame for the planets demise and this climate thing, you and me. Can this be true, no it's a hoax but we are a part of it so that is a little bit true.

> It is not you that is polluting the planet "they" are
> and "they" use your money to do it.
> You do make it possible for "them"
> and therefore are part of the problem
> because you buy into "their" shit stories
> and fill your life with all the toys and things
> "they" say you must have
> while you throw away the unused or broken to pollute.
> All of this is you giving consent
> To their creation
> At the expense and loss of your own

The real problem lies with you and me, all the people together for not informing ourselves of the truth of things and by way of our inaction to stop or reject the controllers greed for power and dominance over you. They have this because you run to spend all the fake money you get for your hard work for them on all the things they say you must have. Shopping, shopping, shopping, your addicted to it and is it all really needed or necessary?
You may well ask.
Stop buying into their story and live your own and then there will be little for them to pollute with and no power to control you.
The controllers and their dependable's and corporate entities are the ones polluting your beautiful planet. You don't have the ability to do the things that are being done but you do make it possible by your silence and compliance.

Some examples:-

+ A rogue section of the military are spraying all the toxic chemicals high in the sky to control and manipulate the weather. This is the climate change they talk of but blame you for. This practice also toxifies the soils so you will find it harder and harder to grow food.
+ Hundreds of ships a year of waste are taken to far lands and dumped and when those lands say no more, they cannot take any

more the ships go to the waters nearby and dump it in the sea to wash up on the shore.
+ There have been war after war and destruction of the people and their land and property everywhere, for what? When you ask this question you cannot find an answer form any reasonable thought, you have to dig into the evil minds and actions of those in control and you will see it is their desire for greed for more and more and you and I are paying the price over and over again for our silence.
+ The vaccination program as stated earlier after compromising everyone by chemical produced food and spreading fake virus's they want you to believe that you will be safe and well again by getting vaccinated by yet more of the toxic shit that caused most of your problems in the first place, come on?
And they now add a microchip and sterilisation to ensure you are safe and under their control.
+ Nicola Tesla, nothing to do with the use of his name today, said when the atom was split that it could be an incredible advancement for humanity but the minds of the controllers would turn it into a destructive force and use it against the people and therefore he would have nothing to do with it. Exactly what happened and they have used your money to amass enough to destroy most of the people on the planet in one sweep. And may I add that this is in the plan for you by them, to be missile targets like all those wars seen on tv or obliterated like the people of Nagasaki and Hiroshima.
+ The testing of these nuclear bombs all over the world has caused so much tectonic destabilisation and more importantly the tests by the USA and France in the pacific were done at weak points and fault lines causing hundreds of miles of underwater volcanic activity which has heated the ocean by 4C+ causing weather instability.
+ The purposeful destruction of the rest of the nuclear power station in japan when the earthquake hit and slightly damaged one of the reactors, so they could dump millions of tons of toxic waste at sea to dispose of it in disguise. But we see how it contaminates the sea and know it is not just that of the reactor out spill.
Now add your own observations of things they do

You did not do any of this, or did you? So why I ask do you get the blame for it all. As said earlier you are helping this to happen by your buying into the story they tell you and that you think you must live to. Stop helping them to do this by not giving them any more of your money or your silence so you no longer need to accept even a little bit of the blame. Question it all and start saying NO.

There is stuff we, as humanity must stop and this is the contamination of the earth, not carbon reduction but the chemical toxification of land, sea and sky, mass drilling and even worse fracking, nuclear testing, bioengineering, especially climate control and of course the constant wars, as it's probably had about enough of us already. If we continue toxifying as we are today, it may just shake like a big shaggy dog and throw us off. I think we are close to this happening should this continue.

In fact if you look at all the flooding, forest fires, melting of the ice, volcanic and seismic activity increase, high winds and exceptional storms and strange happenings, you will see that this is not climate change but climate manipulation and the actions of some very sick people. The military industrial machine has been testing toxic germ warfare and manipulating climate with chem trails, scientifically called bio or geo engineering and frequency (HAARP) on us all for many years, in fact at least since WW2. This is climate change through weather manipulation using toxic chemical spraying high in the atmosphere and then hit by frequency to manipulate it for rain or drought. But again they want you to think you are doing it while they laugh at your stupidity in believing it. But did you noticed the change in the climate when the whole world went into this ridiculous and tyrannous house arrest of everyone. There was not so many chem trails with few planes about so there was nothing to haarp. The sky's were clear and the planet is already in the cleansing and repair process from all the crap they have been doing to it for so long. Look at what is happening all over the world and you may be horrified or you may be thankful that our beautiful planet has the ability to heal itself.

Incidentally the chemicals used in the weather control geo-engineering are causing so many health issues to us and the planet too. It is killing the plankton and raising the temperatures in the sea, destroying the ozone layer, reducing the oxygen and poisoning the soils, reducing both land and sea ability to supply us with the air and food we need. These toxins kill off 10 times more of the expected number of species to become extinct yearly and this will include you and your family too if it continues as your sperm count is down more than 50% in 50 years along with your health and many other issues. But worst of all is that since this spraying of the skies started after WW2, increasing as the spraying has been increased, dementia is now said to be the no 1 cause of death.

> You are being played and played BIG
> and they are laughing with hysterical excitement at you
> while you torture each other
> and they take and torture your children.

Stop and take out these controllers and their hatred for humanity and all of this will stop, just go away, for you and I will not do these things, we will find ways to work within nature as we must, right.

Do not sit on your thumbs though, now you know what is causing all the estranged and unusual weather for it has become even worse since the lifting of lockdown. Contact your leaders and demand they serve you to have this catastrophic practice stopped. And all the others too, after all you pay them to serve you.
Is this the same sort of crap other civilizations did on mars to destroy its atmosphere and toxify the planet? Although I do not believe that story either but it may apply to other planets. This is a battle that must be won together, or all is lost for everyone.
Put the book down and before you continue, write to you leaders about this demanding that it is stopped immediately.

Stop polluting
There are so many things we would be wise to revise or do differently in relation to the environment, like reducing consumption and thus pollution. The madness of drilling the hell out of our planet to take a substance out of the ground, then burning it and setting it free to pollute the atmosphere. The seemingly endless dumping of all sorts of toxic waste into the ocean and the spraying of toxic chemicals in the skies from airliners. You too can come up with more I know as there is so much stupidity being done today under the shadows of profit and their perceived control.

> All future manufacturing must be waste free
> or fully reusable or recyclable without any toxification.
> It is all possible.

The oceans and the air are the life blood of our wonderful earth without both in delicate balance we cannot survive and thrive.

Ocean Temperatures

Some of the genies are out of the bottle already, of which the powers have already done, and we are already seeing the damaging effects. Take the weather instability everywhere on earth now and know that this is not related to the concept of global warming or climate change but the direct results of geo-engineering of spraying toxic chemicals in the sky by various military groups as indicated before and nuclear blast testing by the good old USA and France in the pacific. The after effects (not even mentioning the possibility of toxic remains) of these tests and the shock waves is the destabilisation of the tectonic plates and the ongoing volcanic activity under the sea, especially in the Pacific ocean, that has heated up the Pacific ocean by 4 to 5C above the normal averages of the past and rising. Which in turn affects the atmosphere. Just a half a degree rise causes instability of the weather. Perhaps they want us to be responsible for this too, so it is covered over and hidden as if caused by the global warming or now climate narrative.

It is imperative to get back, to work with and support nature and not as we are at present contaminating, altering and destroying it.

Regaining the trust of nature

is the only way for humans to survive let alone thrive.

Solar

On a more positive note we could support the introduction of solar Roadways. Solar roads could be used everywhere to supply energy to everyone however at this time storage of the energy for off times still needs further development, but I am sure this too will be achieved soon

Energy

There is solar energy, Fuel cells, earth conditioners, natural generators and even the Hendershot magnetic motor/generator and Nicola Tesla's atmospheric energy capture system and so many more that have been discovered/developed and available to improve humanity but they have been locked down from society by the controllers because the money is in the present technology and controlled by the same few. There is a short list of some 89 inventors that have been killed by the shadow controllers black ops enforcers and all their information and inventions seized and hidden from humanity. And I'm sure there have been many more.

Now there is talk of wireless electricity where they install a small unite by your house and supposedly wirelessly send energy to it. This unit is a small Tesla tower drawing energy from the atmosphere for free and the wireless part is to control it and relaying how much you use so you can pay the power company. Buy the machine outright and remove the wireless transmitter and you will have free energy thereafter. Yet another way control and power is used, and the truth hidden for you so they can continue to profit.

> I believe there will be a renewal of these devices
> and especially the Hendershot magnetic motor/generator
> for it is perpetual motion developing energy
> indefinitely, almost.

There are so many other projects too that work and support nature that you can support the people with them instead of supporting the present big corporate growth economic nonsense where finite resources are used faster than you can say blue, and all that they produce is dead foods and the latest fashion trends.

> You may think they are "cool"
> those dead foods and latest fashion
> but who got you believing that story,
> who is controlling your thinking
> for their benefit, their profit.
> Your loss, of health and wealth

Think that through enough and you will know it to be true, although your ego is probably saying right now that "I think for myself, I do." Just observe that and keep thinking, for it is all manipulation to take the money from your pocket to theirs and you will see they have done a great job of it if you take note of where you are and where the money is today.

Follow the guidance
First follow the guidance above to be healthy, speak up further against all the nonsense of today's big business scams, chemically toxic and GM food, your addiction to keeping up with the latest in image gear for they are killing the soils which kills the food and then killing you and me with the final outcome of killing the planet. The big Pharma and chemical companies are the real danger you face if you wish to survive, for this is changing and weakening your immune and DNA systems, not just the planet.

Governments around the world are now manipulated and
controlled by big business and their bankers
to do the bidding for their Big Business.
When they are supposed to be working for the people
You must stand when others stand
and quietly demand they serve you
with honour, in respect of all
For they are your SERVENT's.

And Stand up for the revitalization of the soils with natural fertilizer's and natures minerals so that you can have nature's own real health without the toxic chemical fertiliser and sprays and additives that are destroying the land and your health today.

Then support all action to have the draconian laws overturned and remove any politician that manipulates the system for personal benefit or gain like buying votes, directly or indirectly or in support of "Big Business" against the people.

Force a change in the law so that any company wanting to pay politicians to do their bidding must put that money into a fund for the people and disclose their biddings.

Politicians must become addicted to serving the people
and not the power of big business as they are doing today.

Consider just WHO are the real culprits in this world of miss-information.
They want you sick and scared, to fit into their sick story for if you are healthy and happy, how on earth will they make their money? How on earth will they control you?

If you do not stand with us and we all act on mass together, humanity may not even make it.

Now there is some talk of ET being involved in all this madness on our beautiful earth but I do not believe they would even need to even if that was their intention. The few demonised forms pretending to be human that have taken the controlling positions over us all have more than enough evil in their psychopathic heads to create such incredible stupidity, segregation, hatred, war, uncertainty and instability that there would be no need for outside influence. Perhaps the aliens have come to try to help us with new technology but it will only be used against us because the controllers only use dark energy for their power and hence the evil outcome we have seen intensify. Surely the aliens would stay away from here because this is such a waring place and if we saw them we would attack them, why would the come for that.
I do believe however, there are what we call aliens but more likely friendly supporters of us, here to help us through and out of this dark control but we must act with this intention too and at least ask openly for their help in this difficult transition.

Remember if you want to go out and demonstrate then police are citizens just like you, are there to serve and protect you but they have been trained to attack you, they are brainwashed that you are the enemy they face not because you are their enemy but you are the enemy of the shadow controllers who they think they work for. Do not kneel or bow when out demonstrating but stand quietly and face off the authority you face but never ever kneel or bow. There is no place in this world for shadow controllers, monarch's, royals or any other supreme leaders or ridiculous ideology as to rule over you as is clearly sung in the uk national anthem. No the elected people are your servants and they are the ones that must kneel and bow to you in service to you. Remember you elected them to serve you, not rule over you.

Now this information is out in the open you can all do something about it
Do not stay in your PLACE as this is what they expect of you.
Do not keep supporting their destructive ideology against you as this is what they want of you.
Do not stay silent as this is the very thing that they demand of you.
Stand quietly and withdraw your support and Speak up when needed, when it is clear that what is being done is wrong.
It is now required of you as you now know this information.
It is your duty to inform others about it and where to find it

> "Freedom is never more
> than one generation away from extinction.
> We didn't pass it on to our children in the bloodstream.
> It must be fought for, protected,
> and handed on, for them to do the same,
> or one day we will spend our sunset years telling our children
> and our children's children
> what it was once like in the United States
> where men were free." – Ronald Reagan

And throughout the world

> YOU HAVE A RESPONSIBILITY, YES YOU
> Here On this Earth
> To walk and support the path of Human progress
> One small step each day takes you a lone way
> And even further
> when we all step together
> PLEASE BEGIN   NOW

As Charlie Chaplin said in his last movie,

> The misery that is upon us, the passing of greed
> the bitterness of those that fear the path of human progress

Watch and listen to his important message

<u>Charlie Chaplin - Final Speech from The Great Dictator</u>

check it out - you may need to use a VPN for some places have
blocked it for copy right reasons, allegedly.

> This is a battle
> A secret world war against the darkness
> That must be fought
> That we must win
> Or all may be lost for humanity
> May we fight and fight hard
> To win our sovereignty
> Our freedom our liberty
> And may this be the last war
> We need to fight
> The last battle
> Your voice and vote matters
> We must fight and win
> For the love of humanity

HW conclusion additional notes
This is an added note to the book and a republish, due to the place we find ourselves.
The world has gone mad and the Mad Screaming Mis informers, the media (MSM) is in full mass hysteria and propaganda mode with the latest covert action against all of us. When the facts do not fit with their narrative they disregard the facts and push even harder on their narrative. Another new cannon pointing at you to bring you to your knees in fear so you will submit to more draconian controls. This is tyranny against the people, you and me for when fear is used to control you, you know your government is not serving you but the shadow controllers who are pulling their little puppet strings.
Although I have been endeavouring to enlighten you gently in this book about Shadow controllers and their dark wishes which you are now experiencing first hand with this present covert action against you, and please do not take my word for it. I ask you to wipe aside your fear and present bios that will hold you from understanding the truth of what you are seeing unfold out before your very eyes. How close are we to being pushed over the cliff of no return, or through the gates of hell yet again and slavery for the few that are left after their killing frenzy, very close.
Why do I stress the point that you wake up to what is going on against you and how does it relate to your health?
Your freedom, sovereignty and safety has a direct relationship to whether you can be healthy and remain healthy. Without them you have no chance to remain healthy for long.
However, awaken now to what is actually happening and we can stop this together and then experience the new energy as it rolls in.

The choice is collective and must be achieved together.

Do not just follow what you are being told
Think about it and Question everything, even your own thinking, do your own research to inform yourself, to raise your awareness and your consciousness

Do your own research on:
1.   What is being said or done and by who.
2.   What will they gain from what they say and do.
3.   Who and what is behind the person saying or doing and what is their gain.
4.   To understand what is the truth you will need to 'HEAR' from your heart what is said. Is it love or fear?
5.   For if it is full of catastrophe, fear, trouble and panic. [e.g. as with the lame scream media] you will know there is an ulterior purpose against you.
6.   Does what you hear sound like it is told for the benefit of all the people? Sometime it does till you hear the underlying message of fear.
7.   Listen from the heart -Trust yourself for you will know the truth when you listen from the heart for you will feel the love in the message even if the message is negative.
8.   No message of with love you know it is not a truth for the people but a suppression of you for control.
9.   Watch for message's of uniform control, like vaccinating everyone or keep your distance and ware a mask. They serve no useful purpose at all, but control of you. Take the mask, the simple mask, it removes your individuality, your esoteric self and symbolises you all as robots in submission of possession, a ritualistic manipulation of control over you. To ware a mask removes self and simulates you in character of the act in which you play, don't do it.

Vaccination is out as stated earlier remedies/solutions are what is needed and as for the stupidity of social distancing it is to keep the human love connection separated so we cannot come together in our power. When two or more are gathered together in unity a third force is activated. This brings great fear to the dark controllers. It is also so their tracking cameras can get a better look at you eye print.

When the media has more than 20% coverage on any one subject you know that there is an agenda being fulfilled behind this that will not be good for humanity. I believe this is a drawing down of the curtains to keep you in darkness. These agendas are another step, or leap in this case, to further the power and control of the few invisible controllers behind the visible leaders of almost every country on this beautiful earth. You may be saying that I am talking conspiracy theories and I say there is no such thing and that is what you have been coerced to believe when the truth is being discredited in such a way. You would also be wrong because it cannot be a theory, because it is actually happening. And the Conspiracy is actually against you, so sit up and be alert, unless you are one of the sick conspirator's.

I ask you, is the lame scream media acting in a rational way in response to this so-called crisis. Are they playing the game of who is infected? One would think so from the disappointed tweets of how few are dying, so much so they are manipulating the numbers so everyone dies from this flue and nothing else, which you know is not true. Are they keeping the narrative of panic and fear alive with 100% constant coverage of just one subject and is there nothing else going on in the world, absolutely nothing? Well it would seem so, but you know this is just not true as there are always other things going on.

When you look at the world today you will think it has gone out of balance and this has caused strange things to happen to the people. So divided, in conflict with each other pitching race and place and anything else against each other. Although this is what is happening it is not the people creating this even though it may eco the sentiment they feel about things. In truth you and I are united together against the real divisive actors, the shadow elite. All of this division comes from the shadow controllers bought and paid for. Projected in the media and with a few paid agitator's can stir the emotions of the masses with ease for the masses are becoming aware that things are not right and they want to support what is right so they join in and get caught up in the frenzy of it all. And its all about power for the shadow controllers to get in their dependable's to rule over you. If we look back a history you will see, this is exactly what the Nazi and Hitler did to gain power and you know what followed that. This will not be any different if they get in power. To them its all about power over you and all the time they should be servants to you.

All of this unrest is part of their greater plan to reduce the population to just a few to serve them in the hell they plan to create. They have a problem though for all the wars and conflict have not killed enough and all of the contrived flues whatever they have called them from the Spanish flue which actually started in America to today's [plan-demic] corona flue so called virus has not worked as they planned. Yes each one takes out a few but their plan is billions dead so what's next. Create enough fear In every one so they will beg for a vaccination to protect them but it will not. If they cannot get you one way they will another so in the so called protection, which we all know is not possible, there are many added chemical's to attack your system and if the recent vaccination spree by bill gates in Africa is anything to go by possible hormones to effectively sterilise or at least abort a new born. A much better way to reduce the population for them, you not having any more kids. In less than 70 years there would be very few left. Perhaps this has already been randomly trialled with all the people having difficulty bearing children today on top of all the other contaminants affecting us today and I have not even mentioned the effect on your spiritual being and development.

I have told you before that this sound like fiction but I can assure you I could not make this stuff up, I am just telling you what these very sick people have planned and are creating for you.

Although this is all planned in secret they get your elected servants to make it happen against you while you pay for it in your taxes. This has been what they call normal for a long time but is so insane that its hard even to explain. It so insane that the best analogy I can relate it to is a western style Russian roulette, to throw a few boxes of bullets into a big bonfire at a celebration party and everyone standing around it watching and waiting to see who survives. Have you all gone mad or are you sleep walking into non-existence.

> ## You are being played
> ## and the media is at the forefront of it.

But why you may well ask?
Why would they do this to themselves. They are just puppets having their strings pull from above, for now dependable's. The bit I don't get is their lack of understanding that when the string pullers have finished with you and me they will go for them next and then they too will become expendable. Interesting would you say? They

must be really asleep or the controllers have something big on them and the string pullers think they are Gods so whatever they do does not matter for all life is theirs to play with.

Now there is no point in me telling you about all the evil of drugs, dirty money, People trafficking especially of young girls and children for their perverted sex and sacrifice, yes I did say that, sacrifice. Nor is there any point in me telling you about the cartels of the world vying for power and control over you, their corrupt money system and corporate control over 99% of all big companies, how their greed is so out of control, how they plan for your destruction so they can gain from it. Yes this all sounds way out there and it is for our simple human thinking but it is true and there really is no point me telling you as you will not listen or even believe because you must go on a discovery and learn for yourself. I just write as they are behaving and I cannot do anything else as I have been tasked to lay out things as they are, for you to see enough to open your eyes and find out for yourself. Also, I can tell you that if you do know the full truth you will not be able to sleep properly for weeks, for some of it is so horrific. So far beyond your normal human mind which is connected by love, believe me I recommend you search a little, enough to verify what is put forward here and then do what I discuss in the next paragraph. There is no point in us all not sleeping, now is there.

While you are at a standstill and waiting for some sort of outcome or if it has passed somehow, I ask you to reflect on what your life has been about, pay attention to how you felt and how you feel right now. I know it may feel like you have been pushed off a tall cliff and you are just floating in limbo waiting for the crash. Well in a way this is exactly what has happened to everyone. We are all floating in limbo so let us hold hands, visually for now, and create a unified force. Breath deep, let your mind go, as you calm, your frequency will rise and this will bring you peace, love and compassion. Just unplug from all the madness out there for a while and with calm, reflect on what you really want. Start perhaps by asking aloud for Sovereign freedom for all with the removal of the evil planners and doers trying to remove this from you
Start thinking about what sort of life you want to have when this is passed. It will pass but what is at the end of it will depend on you

and all of us together, our choices, our collective decisions now of what we will consent to, agree with and even support.

I personally will not consent, agree or support anything put forward from their plan as it is evil beyond most human thinking. I will not feed the black hole of doubt and fear nor agree to the controls of psychopaths. I will not spend any more of my money on buying the crap they sell to keep us poor and make them rich. May I suggest you do the same? If that is "normal" I do not want it.

Remember from history it is the losers that write the songs while the victors writes the history. Does this have to play out one more time.   Is this why bob Dylan has put out the new song "murder most foul" stating send your brothers we will kill them too. Does this mean they are now running scared themselves?

In a strange way this time of lock down is a gift. A great gift and a timely gift that no others have had available, where everyone is standing still. Think, project and prey your heart preys to manifest a better future for all. Remember we are all in this together and although they have tried to separate everyone, and silence your voice with a mask, those with the right intention are even more unified in spirit. We may be standing apart, but our candles are still shining light on their darkness.

Self-care has a quantum affect and benefit on all others too, stay calm and stay bright and remember, if you are human,
   ALL LIFE MATTERS.

Remember

Inaction is an action of acceptance in someone else's agenda
so take the action and make a better life now,
Don't ask what others can do for you,
ask what you can do for them
and how you can make a better world for all,

Demand your freedom from the present entrapment
and abuse of us all
What you do does matter, do it now
Its better to be a little early than a minute late
to protect your future
the future of all

#WWG1WGA

I challenge you
to challenge every single thing I put forward in this book
for I know if you have searched enough
you will find it to be the way things are

and in your search, everything in the world today
you will find a story behind their story
that is not for you

12   DECIDE

Recap and Conclusion, keeping on track and What should we Do now?

> What you think and speak
> Changes outcomes
> What you imagine
> And act on with the right intent
> Creates a better world
> Your voice and vote matter

Be the voice of your generation and make some noise
By understanding what Big Business does not want you to know
And Politicians are afraid you will find out.
You get your personal and group power and control back
First off
Can you be confident that what you believe is true,
is actually how it is?
or that you are Right, to believe it anyway
and if it is not, what is your Right position costing you?
The only degree of certainty, is that all, is not as it seems
they say we are in the age of information and technology
If so, it is most certainly not the age of truth
perhaps we are entering the age of awareness
as we come out of barbarism
with fake news masquerading their narrative as facts
One sided and fraudulent and focused only on profit and power
No longer support politicians to enact laws
that force your compliance
Not based on Health or Well Being
or any sort of truth for you and me

Now I'm not saying that everything in this book is true as there is so
much more to know and add but it is as close as I can get with the
information I have gained so far.
In fact, under the official line of things, none of it is true.

Although it is based on 30 plus years of research, experimentation and observations of how things are, not just my own.
 Of me and friends and willing participant's working on every aspect to confirm the outcomes suggested.
Now I ask you too, to Question and observe and decide for your self

A vital first step is to consider what you believe and are thinking, is it helping you achieve what you desire or does it focus on helping others around you. Not your family, I mean your boss or big corporate, the money system. Remember you can be "Right" or you can be healthy, wealthy, wise and have love in your life. However you must have your thinking in balance first.

Then consider what you are Eating and Drinking, before you have a problem with your health and if you already do have health issues then act fast.

Just because you are looking healthy on the outside
Does not mean you are not breaking down on the inside

What is in your hand or close by ready to be in your hand to lift to your mouth and suck or stuff down your neck. Whatever it is, it is the cause of your health condition you are in today or are leading to. If you are fat today, then it is the crap you are eating or choosing to eat and the craving it gives you, that is the cause of you being fat. Until you change your mind and choose differently, you will just get even fatter, sicker and die years before you should.
You do not want that, really, do you?

Also
BE CAREFUL OF THINKING
THAT ALL FOODS ARE YOUR FRIEND
THEY ARE MOST CERTAINLY NOT IN TODAY'S WORLD.

Again, LOOK at what's on your fork, spoon or in your hand that you are about to stuff into your mouth or pour down your throat?

12 DECIDE

Now look at your condition, your size, your shape and how you feel and know that what you are about to stuff into your mouth is the cause of your condition.
If it makes your brain crave it, it will be because your stomach hates it. Only with time following what your stomach loves and only eating that, will your brain stop the cravings for shit food and start to calm and love you too. As a side note this applies to things like smoking, drinking and other addictions too. Remember your gut and brain work together in support of each other so love and respect them both properly so they can return the love so desired.

Start with removing - All heat-treated oils, Refined Sugars, Wheat and Dairy products, then you will find if there are others to remove. Keep adjusting and listening to your body as different things may affect you today than the ones of yesterday. Until we choose to grow food with nature, It will be an ongoing process removing the offenders and finding the supporters, when you do this, joy will fill your body.
If you are overweight or having health issues is it all in your head.? Well not quite but the story you are telling yourself may perpetuate your issues. Go back to the whisper chapter on your head and begin to love yourself again, give yourself a break for it is the information you have been told and gathered along the way that is bad and against any possible chance of you getting success in almost anything let along health. Rewrite the story with selflove and live to it and everything will be different.

Improve your story every day
and your health, wealth and wisdom
will improve and grow with it.

Your genetics, except in some very rare cases, influence your outcome directly only a very small amount, possibly 10% or perhaps even less. The real issue is cultural. In other words, your genetic makeup may influence the outcome a little on its own, while its your lifestyle and cultural habits that influence your outcome and then this affects your genetic regeneration a huge amount especially if your genetics are susceptible to that influence. If you have genetic lack of resistance, then this may cause an Immune inadequacy response. This is especially true in the case for the next new-born when the mum is compromised as you all are today in the western world this will pass to the next born.

Your lifestyle and cultural habits are the key to where you are right now, and this especially applies to how you treat and feed yourself.

Even more important is what you are doing to your kids (if you have them) because young lives are affected far greater and far faster as their delicate structures are still in development.

If you take this a step further, if your own health is compromised and you conceive a beautiful little cherub then how are you going to develop this baby inside you into a healthy child. It will come out compromised already with none of the balance from mum to give it a real chance. It will have all the imbalance from its mum and start life with a very weak immune system and be even more affected by the foods you will then proceed to feed it.

Each generation becomes more and more compromised with a weaker and weaker immune response ability.

To fully understand the present situation you are in regarding your health you must look at history, where we were and what has changed to get us all to where we are today. I have endeavoured to puts forward some of the most significant changes and the effects of those changes on us all, and what you can do immediately to help improve your health.

The good news though is that with this shut down and time to reflect we have a chance of a reset to a better world. Not the un's sick "new world order" reset but one of sovereignty and nature.

May we work on this together to make it happen and there is no place for the so-called supreme leaders or elites for their minds are filled with hatred, destruction and greed.

This is not the complete solution; it is just the beginning and any information or ideas that you can add that improve your health and can improve the health of us all will be welcomed.

Pass it forward at HealthWhispers.com   to Add your input.

Thank you with Love from all humanity

The food and chemical producers have a lot at stake in this, for if the real truth gets out, instead of their manipulated story and you spread this real truth as put forward here so enough people stop using their products they will lose their profits. The beasts they have grown into will die. This is why they keep their lies alive in any way they can and especially by discrediting others.
 And you will know, if they discredit this book and the author of it or suggest a conspiracy, then you know the information is so much closer to the truth than you could have thought possible.

In reality big business and their puppet governments, who were actually elected to serve you, have grown into huge monsters and now both monsters are out of control, addicted to money and power and scheme against you for more.
We must all work together as one, you and me, to stop these monsters ceasing control of everything in our lives including the sovereign you. This unfortunately is very close to happening.

Your voice for freedom must be shouted again, loud and clear.
There is no need to protest in the streets, riot and damage property, get beaten by the simple-minded police who are just another instrument, grunts doing the dirty work of the controllers.
What you must do is simple but as so many will say, it is not easy. The answer is to withdraw your support and stop feeding the monsters and confront your servant in government to be your servant. It's that simple, stop giving your money to anyone that does not support you and your family and the people, because they are using your money to go around the world destabilising and killing the people in far places for their business partners to profit. Beware you could be next although I think it is already happening throughout the west too only in a different format, at least for now. If you have watched the films from "Clockwork Orange", random acts of violence in the community, "The Hunger Games", "The Patriot" and "Loose Change", the way things will be and you will be treated when they get control, "The Huntsman", the taking of your children, "Avatar", the truth of your spiritual extension and that they will do everything possible to destroy your ability to connect or interact with your inner power, the "Matrix" is there next major goal to use nano technology to chip you and manipulate you as if you are a robot in their control, human influenced by AI and many,

many more with every film, filled with violence and building to a frensy of violence of late so you will think that violence is the normal way of humans, it's not, it is their way and their story.
It is mind control so you will be against one another. Remember their goal is to kill 9 out of 10 of us any way they can and control the rest, those left as robotic slaves and for sick sacrificial rituals. Watch them and you will know they have told you what they have planned for you and your children for it is already happening. Beware.

Truth within fiction and Fiction where you expect truth

Truth told through the movies and fiction in the news

As for those big business manipulators that you want to stop polluting your world, then stop buying their crap, especially the toxic food, drink and drugs and most of all do not buy into their news/smoke screen of the day, put out by the main scream media that just happen to be owned by the very same big business owners that want you to buy into their smoke. It may be even better for us to start our own money system or use crypto's that they have no control or access to, although beware for this too is in their plan. The monster may swing its tail in retaliation when it gets hungry for money but if you all, together, just stop feeding it, it will soon die, and you will be free men and women again for the dark energy can only continue with your support, your feeding it. It's that simple.

There Is No Point in Reading This Book
And Not Taking Action on the information.
The journey to your spiritual understanding,
to wisdom,
is not an outward path
but an inward focus

-

The same applies to your health.

Do not go out to big business, the media, your doctor, the next latest Fad Diet for your health. First focus inside to the messages your body is telling you all the time.

12 DECIDE

Life is far too short to be ramrod by others for their gain at the expense of your health, wealth and dreams.

Just remember to ask yourself
"Whose life am I living?" and "Am I living on MY purpose?"

When you are acting from a place of personal empowerment, compassion, fairness and truth, it will be right for you and also for those around you in the long run so why not speed it up and achieve what you require -   sooner rather than later
WHY WAIT?

When you do take action on the information within this book you will be surprised and pleased to find success manifesting in other areas of your life too, once your health improves. Stick to it and you may even find yourself singing or whistling as you walk because you feel so good.
Shake your body and feel your sexy self again, wonderful.

To recap and if you like Rules then these can be your Rules
 If you don't like rules then choose to start today In whatever way you can for better health.
12 step introduction:
1. Enlightenment of your Mind and Intention for a better story.
2. Be positive and live in gratitude, it's better for your health and for everyone around you. Think more of yourself and speak more carefully, more positively, more creatively.
3. Inspire yourself by finding and Removing the Offenders
4. Offenders are stressing and compromising your body. Stop them as fast as you can so your body can repair and calm.
5. Regenerate by Eating Your Supporters
6. Supporter's bring you energy and feel-good feeling calm without hunger, cravings, ravings or envy.
7. Enthral with Fine Tuning your body bio
8. Keep adjusting in small ways, small steps every day in everything you do to get to the best results.
9. Invest in your understanding of Intolerances
10. The Serious Offenders are killing you faster than you know? Keep away from them for an amazing uplift.

12 DECIDE

This includes unhappiness, misery and negativity so be as
happy as you can and laugh every day.
11. Impact your progress with Exercise
12. Do it – use it or lose it, Mind, body and soul.

Taking it further
Your future can and will be more interesting and even exciting.

Talk to your body, with love and gratitude for it to be healthy and
repair the things that trouble you and be amazed at the progress
you make over time with your health. Remember It can take time to
repair just as it took you time to get to where you are.

The internet is a physical manifestation of human future psychic
abilities to interact with each other and accessing the collective
consciousness. It started with a connection then a letter (email)
then a paragraph (FB) then a snippet (twitter) then a picture
(Instagram) and so on. This gives you access to all knowledge in
ways that I believe we all will be able to do through our mind and
body in the near future. Created in the physical to prove the idea to
our linier minds and simplistic human conditioning.

You now know some truths and have opened to other thoughts -
You may believe or not what is put forward here but please
understand it has been brought to you with love to help you.
And do not attack the messenger or you may find you are the
cause or the controllers have the strings tight on your mind control.
There may also be a mistake or two and I'm sure if you are in your
"Right" position you will want to correct or condemn, don't do it, for
this book is about and for YOU and they don't really matter.

I ask you again and again do not take my word for it, research and
find for yourself and remember to act on it or you will not know it at
all.   Do not stop now.

Not to act is to risk everything.

One small step every day will take you a long way
and spread the word speedily and quietly too - shush

Remember
The Big Business has no interest in your health only what is in your purse or pocket. MONEY.
Just like the advertising manipulation of fashion, you are seriously misled over food and health.
Both their food and message are body and mind toxification.
It is all a lie to suck you dry of your wealth and your health.
While you get addicted to and distracted by all the toxic rubbish Big Business promote as healthy, the money gets sucked out of your pockets into their vaults and your health goes with it.
Understand this and STOP IT.

With today's controllers,
The so called ruling elite
power is always taken
And never given
They are the ones that have it backwards
But we have allowed this to happen.
With our silence and compliance.

No more
Now we "the people" demand they step aside
For those willing to give the power to the people
to never take it
or advantage of it
for they are your "Servants"

Do it for what you will become

Why oh why can you even imagine
that you are not affected by the practices of today.
Like the Bees, the impact on you
is showing to be just as severe
As thousand die daily, silently and painfully.

You eat at the end of the food chain
where all the contaminants gather.
What they do, out there, hits YOU, in here
They give you fake medicine to fix it

They think you are stupid
blind, deaf, gullible and easily led
Perhaps you are all of them
Or are you just asleep

Time to Wake up, dear human
join together for better methods,
Or you and the rest of humanity
may be subject to a dramatic decline

Forget global warming, or the next ice age
you'll be long dead, dead food and suppression
watch your "Right" position, for what it is costing you
don't wait for them, to make your life hell

Are you doing it by choice
predictive programming, or is it by force?
What is your assignment here anyway?
to keep the game of life infinite

then wake, stand and speak
it is your Right; it is your domain.
How are you living your own plan
Your own dreams?

No need to join their new world order
of control and forced occultism
or fight against them or even involve witchcraft
or initiate anything else of their evil creations

For when their message of hate and greed
and centralised control is understood
and no longer acceptable by you, or engaged by others
the correction to a better reality begins

Survival of humanity in its beautiful life statement
quietly withdraw your support from all unethical organisations
including governments not servants, of the people
don't have life leaning on you, lean into life.

Life, the only real precious thing you have
your health your freedom, far too important
to leave to the covert kingdoms and politicians
or big Pharma, bad

Everything has a cycle
the present system already expired
the world is on fire for a better way,
look, you see it, all over
the more it's resisted the faster it goes

melting ice and brimstone, fire and floods
earth changes and quakes
our world is cleansing, you must too

Share this information quietly
till it can be shouted from the hill tops.
no big demonstrations, no protests, no unnecessary dying
Simple, withdrawing your interest,
your support of them

Stop buying their smokie stories
stop buying their crap
Keep your money in your pocket
to empower yourself

Just Smile at them as you walk past their doors,
on your way to a better supplier
where you can buy nature's own quality produce
And rebuild your Health along with your Wealth.

Don't be disheartened
if this sounds impossible
for in its place
something beautiful is coming

no matter how fast they run
the truth is always a few steps ahead
no longer stealing your ball or stopping your flame
no power to control, pressure, isolate, or assassinate.

Your action is needed
Will you run and hide
To your cave of fear and despair
Or will you stay and fight this one last fight

In support of us all
What will you choose?
Stand tall or Hide
Become what you are meant to be

no harm must be done
life is a Present
new cycle, new energy already surrounds you
shining the truth, with love

How close are you to nature?
Slow, to its natural pace and beauty
Lay on the ground, for its energy
Stare upon it, for its love is returned

You are not alone
love surrounds, fills and supports you
Feel it, for it is with you
and so are we

I'm making my ripple
you make yours
together we will change our world
for the better,
One small step from you and one from me
Creates a giant leap for mankind
prepare for the new.

The earth has a much greater impact and connection
To our existence than we know.
Our living planet of abundance

And who said we are alone in the universe
Those that are afraid you will know
Your power within
And shine your light on their darkness

RESOURCES

We have not included resources for this guide other than the few mentioned within, for the following reasons.

According to the official line, nothing in this book is true, so therefore there will be no resources to find, right, even though you will find it exactly the way things are when you do your own research. I have pulled the curtains back and shown some light on the truth, its now up to you to draw them back further and do your bit too

When you do your own research, you will find all the information is available to you provided you are tenacious and persistent. As I have revised this book over the years there has been more and more information coming out even in the main fake news press, usually hidden in the back pages and possibly missed or still confusing you I'm sure, but some are getting closer to the truth of things. Keep watching and observing based on what you have learned here, and you will see the trend is changing for the people.

We are also finding that the shadow controllers are running scared and blocking as much information that does not match the story they want you to believe so you may only see the story put out once in the press and then it is removed, because if you know the truth it will affect their profits and their position of power, so please be aware of this too. I was blocked from FB for putting out this information. It's not what the CIA wants for its shadow controllers and big corporate.

Health Whispers will put up and keep up as long as it can a resource where you can find links to some research and knowledge to get you started.
healthwhispers.com

Check out the movies for you may see them differently now

Remember truth within fiction and fiction where you expect fact,

Look around you, be alert and watching in your local area and let us know what you see and what you can do to change things for the better, thus giving ideas for others too.

As sad and distressing as some of the info in this book is, if the learning and tips help you understand things and improve your health for the better and you would like share what you learned and to know more from others about how to continue the process of great health ideas then come together at   HealthWhispers.com
Your experience and learning are of value to us all, "Together"

The intention of this information is to inform you and help you to a better life so that you can then help others to better lives too

Is this enough? most certainly not.
This is not the whole solution
 it is just the beginning, the first baby steps,
To make it better we need YOU, your action too
For we all must come together in sovereign collaboration.

RESOURCES

The last word   :)

Is this enough
No way
It is just the beginning
For humanity to do it differently
To do it better

New thinking is required from
Outside our singular, linear spectrum
receive the knowledge
and inspiration of quantum love
from the many, external, entangled continuum

Remember
Keep up the action
your voice and vote matter
Together, We Can.

Create now for the new and better future
No new normal
For the future is now

Calm your mind
Settle in, to the divine you
Honour and Love one another
Shine your light, so Humanity can see
Live,   in Love and Compassion

To your renewed and wonderful life.
To us all

RESOURCES

9 798683 444471